ABC OF
OTOLARYNGOLOGY

ABC OF OTOLARYNGOLOGY

HAROLD LUDMAN MB, FRCS

Consultant Surgeon in Otolaryngology
King's College Hospital, London

and

Consultant surgeon in neuro-otology
National Hospital for Nervous Diseases, Queen Square, London

Published by the BMJ Publishing Group
Tavistock Square, London WC1H 9JR

British Library Cataloguing in Publication Data
A catalogue record for this book is available from the British Library

First edition 1981

Second edition 1988

Third edition 1993

ISBN: 07279 0765 4

Typeset in Great Britain by Apek Typesetters, Nailsea, Avon
Printing and Binding by Eyre & Spottiswoode Ltd, London and Margate

Contents

ACKNOWLEDGEMENTS

The photograph of an operating microscope (p 12) is reproduced by permission of Carl Zeiss (Oberkochen) Ltd; that of an audiometer (p 13) by permission of Amplivox; those of spectacles and hearing aids (p 16) by permission of PC Werth Ltd; and that of Hopkin's rod-lens telescopes by permission of Smith and Nephew Medical, Hull. I thank Dr J M Dawson for kind permission to reproduce the radiographs on pages 31, 38, 39, 44, 46, 52, and 53, and Mr J A M Martin, director of the Nuffield Hearing and Speech Centre for kind permission to reproduce the photographs on pages 20 and 21.

PAIN IN THE EAR

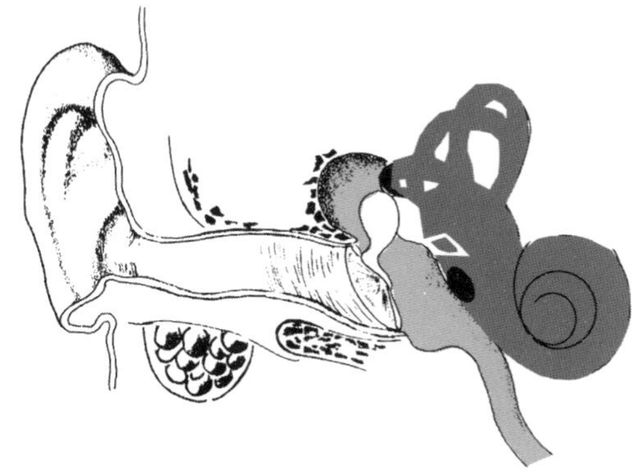

Inflammatory causes of pain in the ear are evident from inspecting the external ear and tympanic membrane. Injuries to the pinna with haematoma are obvious from the history. Perichondritis of the pinna is a rare complication of injury, usually surgical. Infection is caused by *Pseudomonas aeruginosa*.

Acute otitis externa

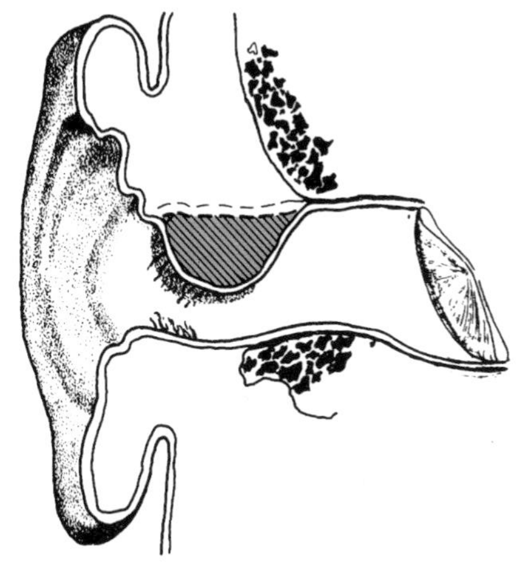

Acute otitis externa may be a diffuse inflammation or a furuncle. A furuncle is a very tender swelling in the outer ear canal (there are no hair follicles in the bony meatus). Hearing is impaired only if the meatus is blocked by swelling or discharge, and fever occurs only when infection spreads in front of the ear, as cellulitis or erysipelas. Tender enlarged nodes may be palpable in front of or behind the ear, but the tenderness is superficial, unlike the tenderness on deep pressure in acute otitis media. The pinna is tender on movement and this, again, does not occur in acute otitis media. Any discharge is thick and scanty, unlike the copious mucoid discharge of middle ear infection. Fungal infections, in particular, cause pain in diffuse otitis externa.

Acute otitis media

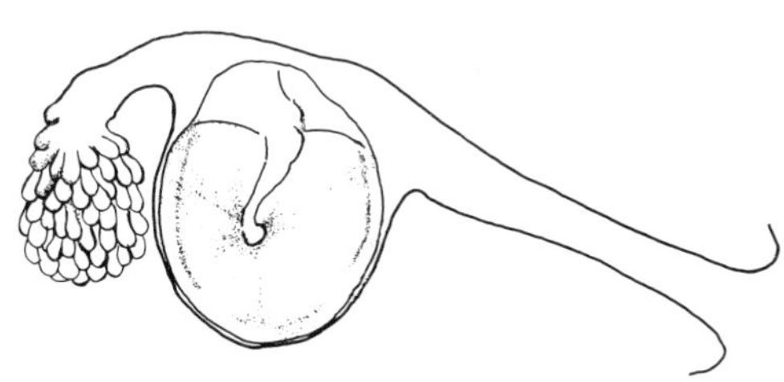

Acute otitis media causes deep seated pain, deafness, and usually systemic illness with fever. The sequence of symptoms is a blocked feeling in the ear, pain, and fever, followed by discharge if the drum head perforates, with relief of pain and fever. Since the whole middle ear cleft is affected there is tenderness on deep pressure over the mastoid antrum; this does not imply mastoiditis. Bacterial infection is usually by *Streptococcus pneumoniae* or *Haemophilus influenzae* in the youngest children. Diagnosis is made by inspecting the tympanic membrane, but this may be prevented by wax or by swelling from a secondary otitis externa. Only if the whole drum is normal and there is no conductive hearing loss can otitis media be excluded. Lymph nodes in front of and behind the ear are never enlarged in simple otitis media.

Acute mastoiditis

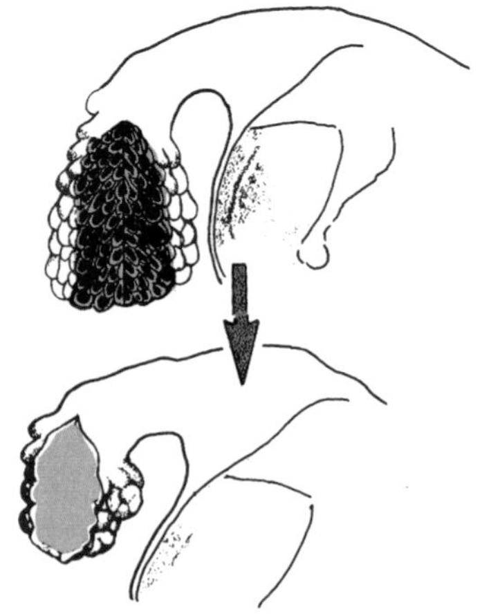

Acute mastoiditis is caused by breakdown of the thin bony partitions between the mastoid air cells—a process that takes two or three weeks. During that time, from the onset of acute otitis media, there is continuing and increasingly copious discharge through a perforation in the drum. If a patient has pain a few days after the drum has been reliably shown to be normal then he or she cannot have developed mastoiditis. The difficulties arise when the patient is thought to have recovered from acute otitis media but the condition has in fact "grumbled" on; sometimes, because of systemic antibiotics, this may have occurred with very little systemic illness. Mastoiditis should be suspected in any patient with continuous discharge from the middle ear for over 10 days, particularly if he or she is feeling "under the weather."

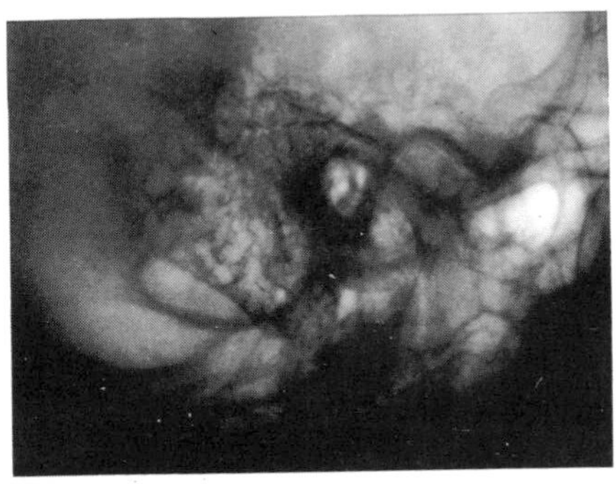

Radiographs of the mastoid may help, but not always. Only if they show a clearly aerated normal cell system can mastoiditis be excluded. The classical appearance of breakdown of intracellular trabeculae is not always seen. Otitis externa may cause haziness of the cell system because of oedema of the soft tissues over the mastoid. The classical swelling behind the ear with downward displacement of the pinna implies a subperiosteal abscess, which is a complication rather than a feature of mastoiditis. A subperiosteal abscess can, by erosion of the outer attic wall, cause swelling in the deep part of the ear canal, in contrast to a furuncle in the outer part. If doubt persists after mastoid radiography surgical exploration may be necessary. High resolution computed tomography is more useful than conventional radiography.

Other complications of acute otitis media

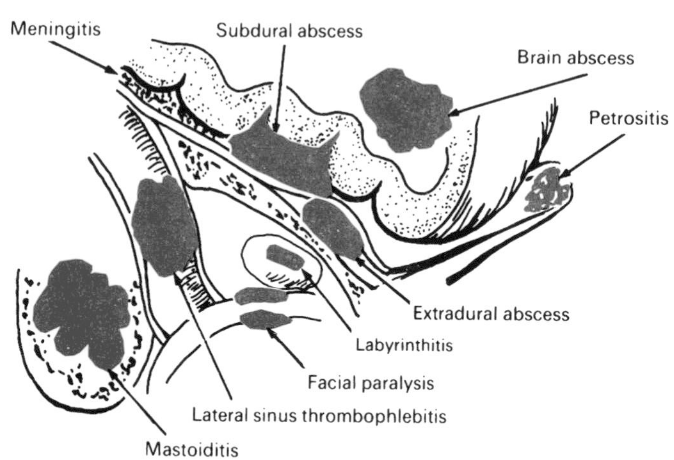

All these are rare. They arise only if infection spreads beyond the middle ear cleft. Complications occurring within the petrous temporal bone are facial palsy, suppurative labyrinthitis, lateral sinus thrombophlebitis; those occurring within the cranial cavity are meningitis, extradural abscess, subdural abscess, brain abscess.

Secretory otitis media (otitis media with effusion)

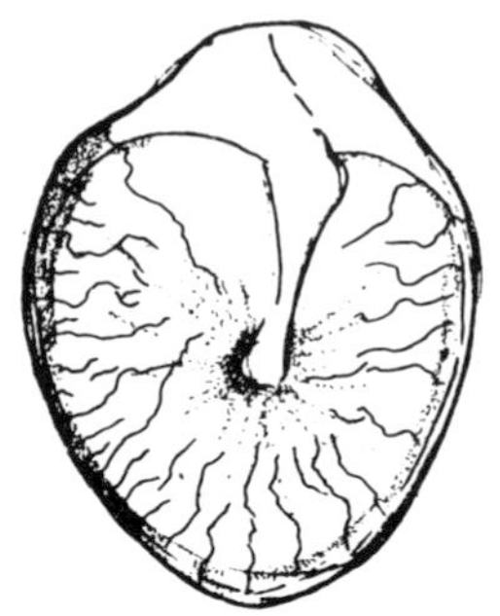

Niggly shortlasting pain is characteristic of "glue ear." The drum looks abnormal because of the effusion. Classically there is injection with noticeable radial vessels, which may prompt a misdiagnosis of otitis media. The colour may be yellowish or sometimes blue. The child is well and afebrile, however, and the associated hearing loss has usually been recognised for some time (see page 22).

Other causes of pain

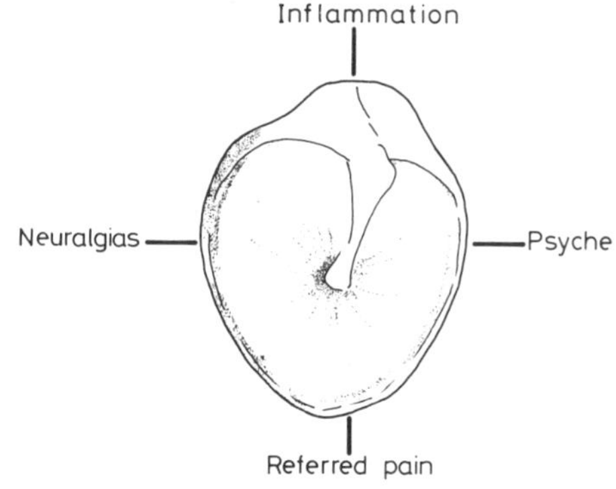

Bullous myringitis is an uncommon cause of severe pain. Viral (probably influenzal) infection causes haemorrhagic blistering of the ear drum and external ear canal. There may be an associated haemorrhagic effusion in the middle ear and it may be difficult to distinguish this condition from otitis media.

If there is no inflammatory ear disease and no disease in sites from which pain might be referred to the ear remaining possibilities are glossopharyngeal neuralgia, migrainous neuralgia, or psychogenic pain. Glossopharyngeal neuralgia is severe lancinating pain in the throat and ear triggered from one or more points in the oropharynx. Tympanic neuralgia produces the same severe stabbing pain with no throat symptoms.

Often no cause can be found for the pain; then it may be due to depression and is often relieved by treatment for that condition.

Referred pain

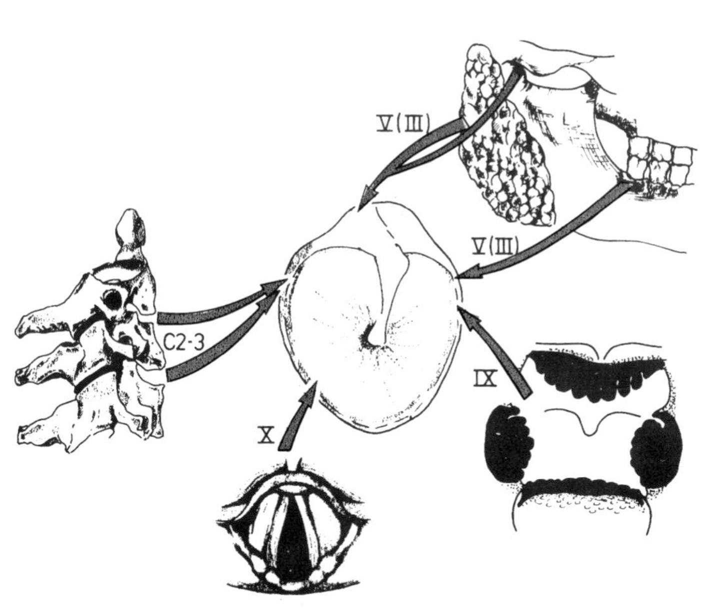

If the ear canal and drum are normal and there is normal movement of the drum on examination with a Siegle's speculum pain is not due to disease of the ear. It is probably referred from territory sharing sensory innervation with the outer or middle ear. Pain may be referred from:

(*a*) The oropharynx (IXth nerve) in tonsillitis or carcinoma of the posterior third of the tongue.

(*b*) The laryngopharynx (Xth nerve) in carcinoma of the pyriform fossa.

(*c*) Upper molar teeth, temperomandibular joint, or parotid gland (Vth nerve mandibular division). Parotid causes are usually obvious: impacted wisdom teeth may not be. Temperomandibular joint troubles often follow changes in bite caused by new dentures, extraction, or grinding down;

(*d*) The cervical spine (C2 and C3). Pain is often worse at night when the head lies awkwardly. Neck support often provides relief, as does a neck pillow under the side of the neck at night.

Treatment of acute otitis externa

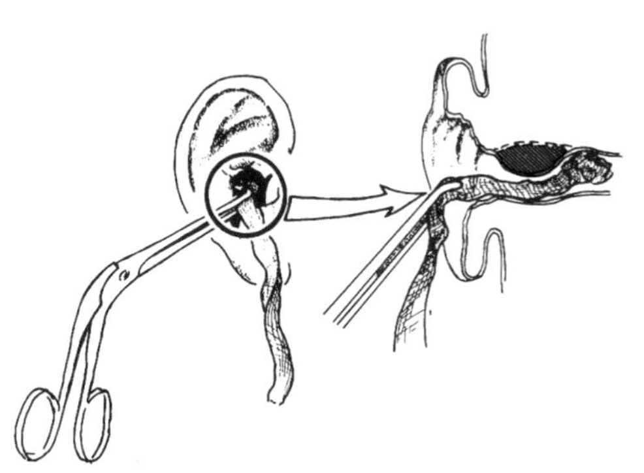

Systemic antibiotics are useful in acute otitis externa only when there is a systemic illness with fever or lymphadenitis, and occasionally in multiple furunculosis. Sometimes meatal swelling must be reduced by inserting a ribbon gauze wick painted with a deliquescent substance such as magnesium sulphate paste or glycerine and 10% ichthammol. The wick needs replacing daily until the swelling has subsided, which is often accompanied by discharge of the core of the furuncle. (Rarely a furuncle may need incision.) Aural drops may then be used—either aluminium acetate to "toughen" the skin or topical antibiotics such as gentamicin, framycetin, or neomycin, combined with steroids. Clotrimazole drops are useful as an antifungal agent. Pain is relieved by systemic analgesics, together with warmth, applied through a hot pad or radiant heat lamp. Recurrent furunculosis may indicate diabetes.

Treatment of acute otitis media

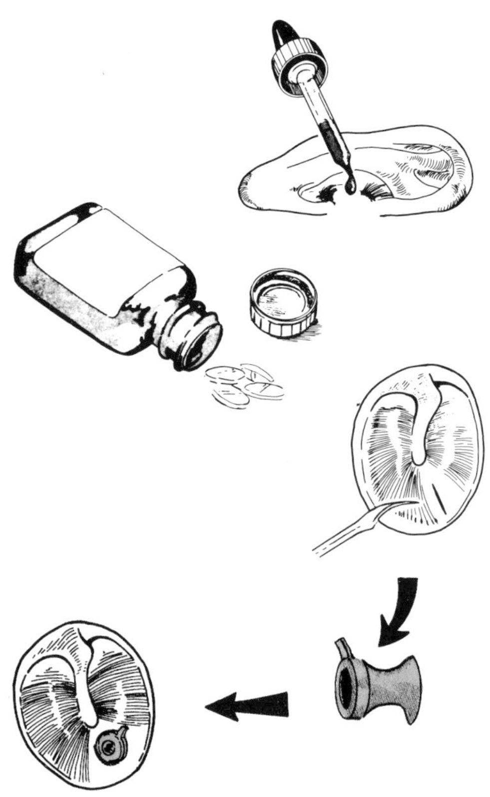

Systemic antibiotics must be used for the treatment of acute otitis media. The commonest infecting organisms are *Streptococcus Pneumoniae*, *Haemophilus influenzae* and *Moraxella (Branhamella) catarrhalis*. The antibiotic of choice, effective against these, is amoxycillin. If β lactamase producing organisms are likely, amoxycillin combined with clavulanic acid (Augmentin) or trimethoprin and sulphamethoxazole may be preferred. Oral administration is advised, even for the first dose, and the drug must be continued for at least five days. Supplementary treatment includes pain relief by analgesics and warmth. Warm olive oil drops may be soothing but nasal decongestants have no proved role. If the drum perforates the ensuing discharge may be cultured, but an antibiotic should be changed on clinical and not solely bacteriological grounds. Rarely the drum may bulge under pressure, without rupture; this would be an indication for myringotomy under general anaesthesia.

Recurrent otitis media may be encouraged by predisposing causes such as persisting middle ear effusions. If this is so then myringotomy with insertion of a grommet is advisable. Occasionally recurrent otitis media may be associated with recurrent tonsillitis, and tonsillectomy might be considered. Similarly, adenoid enlargement and recurrent infection may be predisposing factors, but the role of adenoidectomy is controversial. Without predisposing factors each attack must be treated as it arises. After an attack a return to normal should be expected and confirmed within three weeks.

Otitic barotrauma (aerotitis)

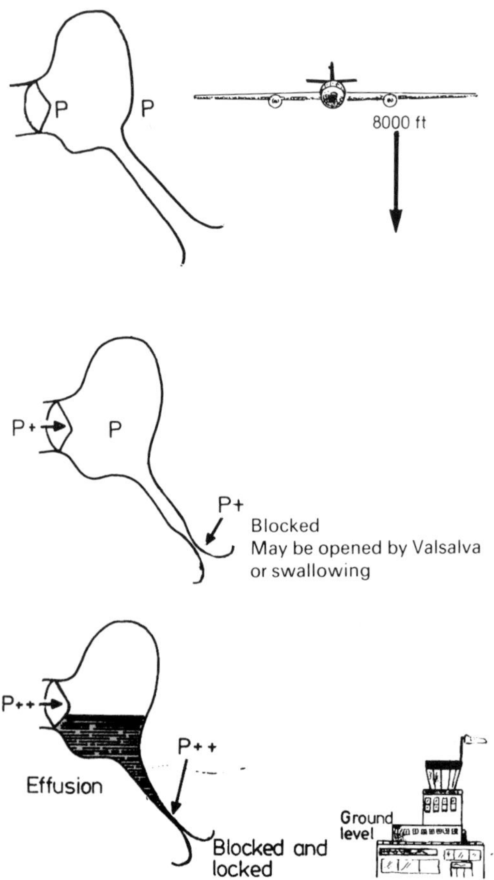

A patient can reduce the risk of aerotitis during descent in an aircraft by not travelling with an upper respiratory tract infection or hay fever. Valsalva's manoeuvre—pinching the nose with finger and thumb and blowing hard down it—should be taught. If this works the patient will feel his ear "pop." If the manoeuvre does not work the doctor should first check that the patient is blowing through his nose and not his mouth. He should ask the patient to blow and then suddenly remove the pinching digits; the ensuing explosion should be through the nose. If he can perform Valsalva's manoeuvre properly the patient should do so during descent as soon as he feels a change in pressure and should repeat the procedure every few seconds whenever the sensation returns; it must not be left until the tube becomes irreversibly blocked. This procedure will prevent barotrauma. Decongestants may also help to clear the Eustachian tube. An antihistamine should be taken the day before and on the day of the flight every six to eight hours. During the flight a spray such as xylometazoline is useful. This should be sprayed into the nose one hour before the expected time of arrival and every 20 minutes thereafter. The first spray should be followed a few minutes later by another, when the anterior part of the mucosa will have shrunk, to allow the droplets access to the nasopharynx.

The only guaranteed way of preventing barotrauma is to insert a long term ventilation tube through the ear drum. This may be advisable for people at risk who have to fly. Patients with middle ear effusions or unresolved otitis media should not fly.

To treat otitic barotrauma the patient needs only analgesics and reassurance. If an effusion persists for more than 10 days a myringotomy may be advisable but need not be considered in the first few days. Systemic antibiotics have no useful role.

Treatment of injury to the outer and middle ear

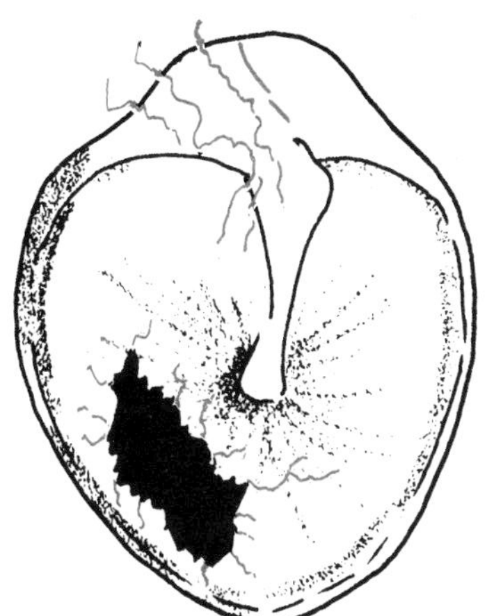

Injuries to the pinna may cause haematomas, which, if repeated and untreated, lead to cauliflower ears. After injury to the outer or middle ear the meatus is usually obstructed by a blood clot. The ear drum need not be examined immediately, but it is wise to assume that it has been perforated and to warn the patient to prevent water from entering. If a foreign body is suspected referral for examination under anaesthetic may have to be considered. With no fever or foreign body antibiotics are not needed, and if there are no complications such as vertigo, facial palsy, or leaking cerebrospinal fluid there is no immediate need to assess the hearing. Perforation of the ear drum or conductive deafness due to ossicular damage may need elective surgery (see page 14), but its discovery can wait until the clot has been extruded and the ear can be examined under the operating microscope. Most traumatic perforations heal spontaneously and operative repair should not be considered until the ear has had six weeks' opportunity to heal.

DISCHARGE FROM THE EAR: OTITIS EXTERNA AND ACUTE OTITIS MEDIA

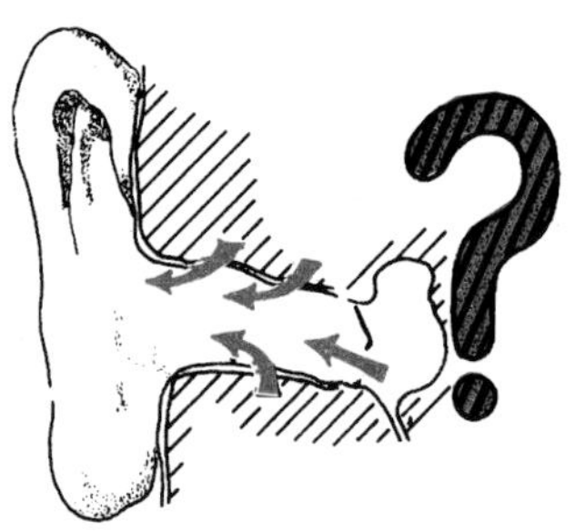

Discharge from the ear occurs in both otitis externa and otitis media. In acute furunculosis and acute otitis media the dominating symptom is pain, which precedes any discharge. Diffuse otitis externa, on the other hand, may present with a thin serous discharge, especially if there is an allergic eczematous reaction. In acute furunculosis the discharge is the thick extrusion of the core of the boil, which consists of necrotic material; there is usually no difficulty in diagnosis.

Acute otitis media

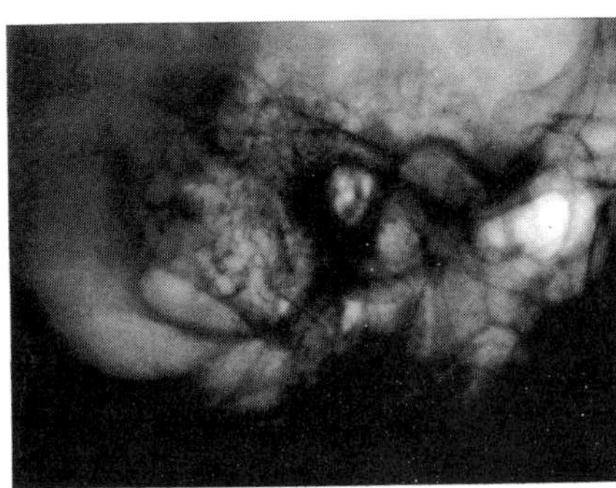

Discharge in acute otitis media, which is profuse and mucopurulent or purulent, occurs only if the drum perforates. It usually stops within a few days and the perforation heals. Profuse discharge persisting for a week or more may indicate the development of coalescent mastoiditis or a reaction of the mucosa of the middle ear to Eustachian tube inadequacy.

If mastoiditis develops continuing discharge is usually accompanied by continuing ill health and tenderness on deep pressure over the mastoid antrum. The systemic signs may be masked by antibiotics. Mastoid radiographs may help: if they show normal air cells with normal bony trabeculae coalescent mastoiditis can be excluded. When uncertain the only safe course is to explore the mastoid.

"Subacute" otitis media

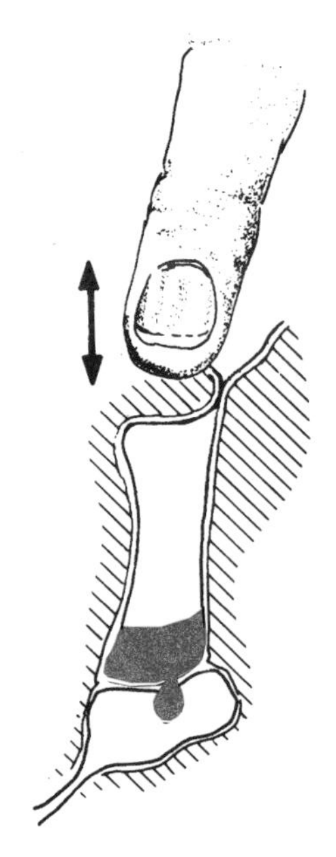

Continuing discharge due to mastoiditis is relatively uncommon. A more common illness is seen when a child is well but still discharges mucopus from the ear three or more weeks after a typical attack of acute otitis media. The pattern may arise when grommets are in place in the ear drum. The reasons include continuing irritation of the mucosa of the middle ear by resistant organisms; continuing infection of the nasopharynx, with secondary infection of the middle ear cleft; and changes in the mucosa of the middle ear secondary to Eustachian tube dysfunction of the kind found in secretory otitis media, with more active secretion than normal. Occasionally an inflammatory, possibly allergic, reaction to the presence of a grommet may cause discharge, and this can be recognised by the appearance of granulation tissue around the grommet, on the surface of the tympanic membrane.

The first step in treatment is to take a swab for culture and to give systemic antibiotics based on the result. After regular gentle toilet to remove infected debris from the meatus, topical antibiotic and steroid drops should be instilled and massaged into the middle ear by pressure on the tragus. In adults radiographs of the sinuses may show evidence of infection that needs treating, or there may be infected mucopus in the nose and nasopharynx. Children should be encouraged to blow their noses to prevent mucus from stagnating and becoming infected. Decongestant nasal sprays should be used after blowing the nose for a *short* period. Systemic antihistamines should be part of the regimen, since allergic swelling of the mucosa around the orifice of the Eustachian tube may be a factor. Provided mastoiditis can be excluded such measures can be used without fear of serious risk for a few weeks. If discharge continues referral is advisable.

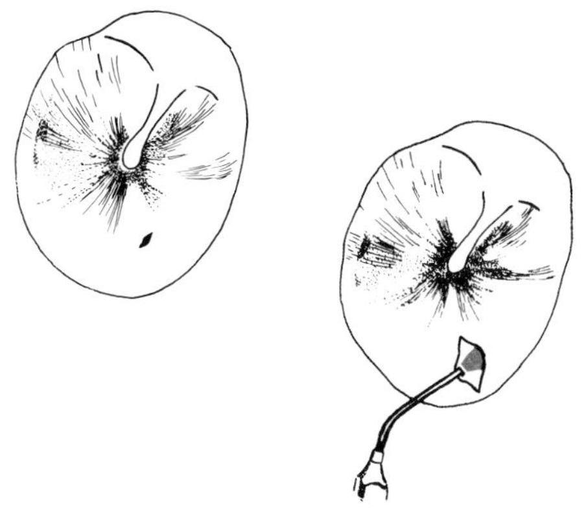

Further helpful measures include removing enlarged adenoids and examining the ear under anaesthetic. The perforation in the drum may be enlarged to improve drainage, while mucoid material can be sucked from the middle ear under anaesthetic. Very rarely continuing discharge may suggest that the mucosa throughout the mastoid air cell system has become secretory. This is an indication for a cortical mastoidectomy to remove the secreting mucosa.

A grommet that seems to be the source of irritation may need removal under anaesthetic.

Chronic otitis externa

Cleaning the ear with a dirty towel is the best way to produce otitis externa

In chronic otitis externa discharge is accompanied by itching, irritation, and impaired hearing. The discharge is often thick, smelly, and composed of infected wax and desquamating skin. The organisms are generally Gram negative. Nevertheless, the ear drum is normal and there is no conductive hearing loss. The condition is almost always bilateral. Unilateral otitis externa suggests middle ear disease: there may be a tiny perforation, not easily visible on examination, and the otitis externa may then be secondary to irritation caused by the material from the middle ear.

Chronic otitis externa is partly due to intrinsic factors such as skin diseases—eczema, seborrhoeic dermatitis, or psoriasis—and partly to extrinsic factors in the form of trauma from cleaning the ears, softening the skin by moisture when bathing, or using a dirty towel. There is no better way to produce otitis externa than to bathe in polluted water and then clean the ear with the corner of an abrasive towel that has collected organisms from other parts of the body.

Treatment

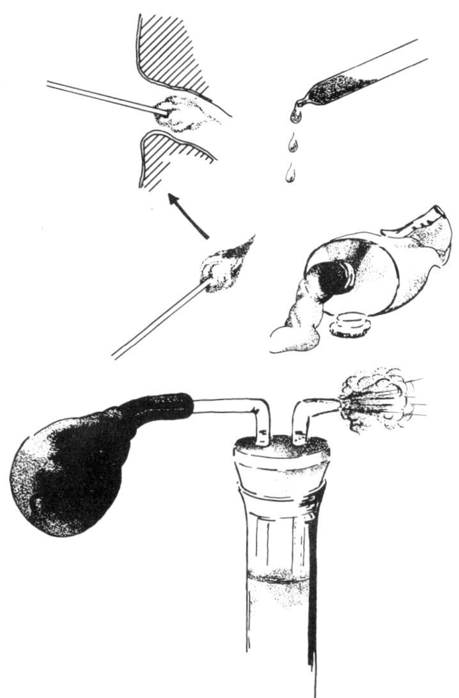

Chronic otitis externa is treated by aural toilet and by instilling topical medication. Careful cleaning to remove infected debris must be done under good illumination with cotton wool on a wool carrier, or by suction under a microscope, paying particular attention to the anterior recess. Provided the drum is intact, gentle syringing can be useful. Toilet should be repeated often—ideally every day; in practice it is usually done once a week. A swab should be taken for culture of fungi as well as bacteria. Useful topical applications include combinations of antibiotics such as gentamicin and neomycin with a steroid. If fungi are present antifungal agents such as nystatin or clotrimazole should be used. The medication may be instilled as drops twice a day, painted on the meatal walls with cotton wool carried on a wick, or insufflated as a powder after toilet.

Systemic antibiotics are unnecessary. Eczematous reactions of the pinna may occur and should be treated with ointment. Allergic reactions to topical applications show themselves by worsening of the condition with redness and profuse watery discharge from the pinna. Topical preparations should not be used for long. There is a case for using drops on a long term basis, but intermittently, say once a week, for patients who readily relapse.

When intrinsic factors predominate cure may be impossible though the condition can usually be alleviated. Rarely subepithelial fibrosis causes gross narrowing of the meatus and the lack of ventilation exacerbates the condition. An operation to widen the meatus is then needed. All patients must be warned to protect their ears from water.

DISCHARGE FROM THE EAR: CHRONIC SUPPURATIVE OTITIS MEDIA

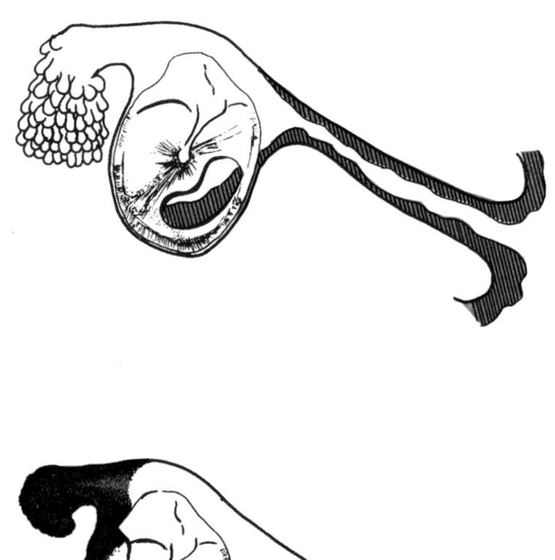

There are two types of chronic suppurative otitis media. Both present with conductive deafness and discharge without pain. In both discharge issues through a perforated drum; but one is safe and the other unsafe.

In the safe variety (tubotympanic or active mucosal chronic otitis media) there is no risk of intracranial life threatening complications. Disease affects the mucosa of the lower anterior part of the middle ear. By contrast, the unsafe variety (atticoantral or active chronic with cholesteatoma) threatens meningitis, brain abscess, and other serious complications. The disease erodes the bone and cholesteatoma and chronic osteitis develop in the atticoantral region.

The perforation in the safe type is central: no matter how large, there is always a rim of drum or its annulus around the edge. In contrast, the perforation in the unsafe variety extends to the very bony edge of the drum, where chronic necrosis of the bone is often associated with the production of granulation tissue. This marginal perforation is usually posterior or in the attic.

Discharge in the safe variety comes from the inflamed and secreting mucosa of the middle ear, and is mucoid. It may be intermittent, with activity provoked by water and by blockage of the Eustachian tube. In the unsafe variety the discharge is often scanty and foul smelling and there are no periods of quiescence. This discharge usually comes from the infected debris accumulating within a cholesteatoma sac. Cholesteatoma is simply skin—stratified squamous epithelium—that has entered the middle ear cleft to form a multiloculated cyst surrounding structures in the attic and extending into the air spaces connected with the mastoid antrum. When the keratin accumulating within the cholesteatoma sac becomes infected the outermost layer of the cholesteatoma sac, which is the basal layer of the skin, starts to erode adjacent bone; therein lies its danger.

Recognition and treatment of safe ears

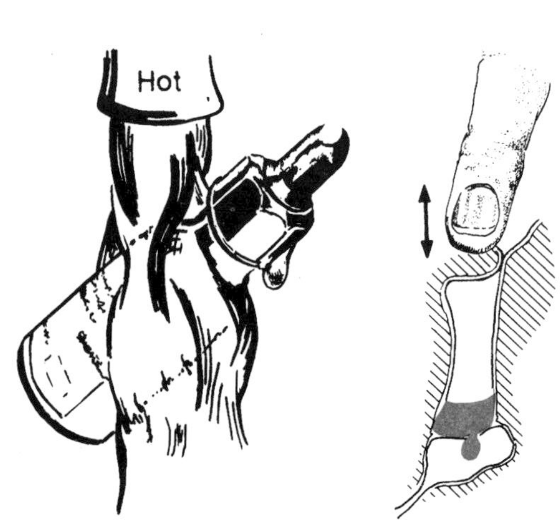

The two types of chronic suppurative otitis media can be distinguished only by carefully examining the ear drum after removing any discharge—ideally under an operating microscope. More than one examination, after reducing surface inflammation with topical treatment, may be needed. Safety is suspect when the discharge smells foul, when there is granulation tissue or a polyp arising from the middle ear or outer edge of the drum, when dead skin or keratin can be aspirated from the middle ear, and when there are symptoms, such as facial weakness or vertigo, that suggest complications. Only when there is a central perforation without any of these features can safety be confirmed.

In safe ears the aim is to dry up discharge, help any hearing defect, and prevent further discharge. Drying is achieved by treating infection or allergy in the upper respiratory tract and by aural toilet to remove infected material. Rarely syringing may help: the best solution, which must be at body temperature, is half strength Eusol in isotonic saline (mix full strength Eusol with equal volume of 2 × isotonic saline). Antibiotic drops containing steroid are useful, and the choice of preparation may be guided by the results of swab culture. The drops must be warmed by holding the bottle under a hot tap, and massaged into the middle ear.

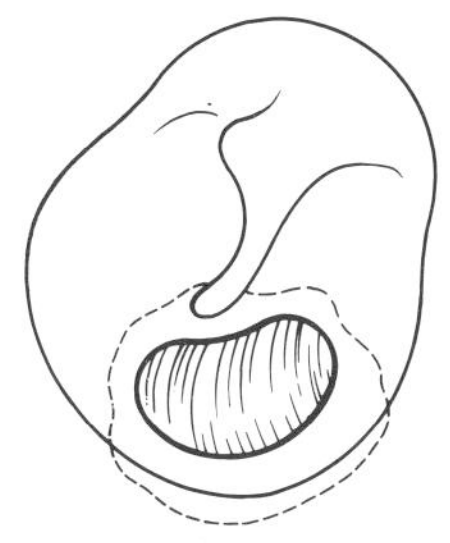

Once the ear is dry, (inactive chronic otitis media) further discharge may be prevented by protecting it from water and promptly treating upper respiratory tract infection or by closing the defect in the ear drum surgically (myringoplasty). Hearing defects can be helped by a hearing aid or by reconstructing the drum and ossicular chain (tympanoplasty).

Treatment of unsafe ears

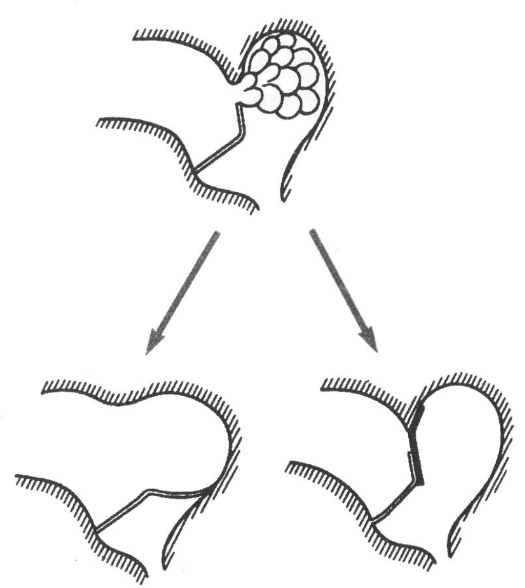

A dangerous ear must be rendered harmless before the problems due to deafness are treated. The aim of the various operations performed—radical mastoidectomy, modified radical mastoidectomy, atticotomy, atticoantrostomy—is to remove diseased and infected bone and leave a smooth wide cavity opening into a wide external ear canal. As the ear heals the cavity becomes lined with skin, which is histologically identical to cholesteatoma, but which excretes its dead squames to the exterior through wide access.

Radical mastoidectomy is an example of this kind of operation. Under general anaesthesia the ear is entered through either an endaural or postaural incision. The mastoid antrum is opened with a drill. As the opening to the antrum is enlarged it extends forward into the attic region of the middle ear. Removing the "bridge" of bone over the aditus ad antrum throws the mastoid cavity and middle ear into one. Disease is removed as the operation progresses. In classical radical mastoidectomy all the ossicular chain except the stapes is removed. The cavity is made as hemispherical as possible, without damaging the facial nerve, labyrinth, sigmoid sinus, or dura. Then the cavity is packed with, for example, ribbon gauze soaked in an antiseptic ointment. Other methods—*combined approach tympanoplasty* or intact canal wall techniques—avoid creating a cavity and try to reconstruct the middle ear mechanism, but at the risk of enclosing residual cholesteatoma.

The complications of unsafe ears are, apart from acute mastoiditis, those of acute otitis media (see page 2).

Discharge from the mastoid cavity

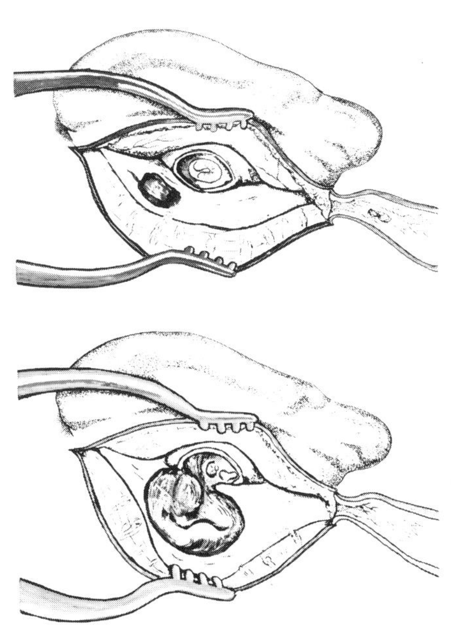

After operation the discharge will continue until the cavity is completely lined with skin—a process that usually takes three months and in some patients is never completed. The reason is that the discharge is exudation (since the body is wet) and the cavity lacks a waterproof lining. Continuing or recurrent discharge is due to anything that prevents or breaks down intact cavity lining. The warm, damp mastoid cavity is inhospitable to healthy skin. Conditions for healing are best when operation creates as small a cavity with as wide an opening to the external meatus as possible. Even then some patients cannot form a healthy lining. Infection of discharging exudate may be a reason for this. The discharge becomes infected with Gram negative organisms from outside or from the nasopharynx; the infected material prevents skin from healing, by its inflammatory action and by producing granulation tissue that cannot be covered by epithelium and that occludes poorly drained pockets of infected material.

During the early postoperative period the ear, protected by gauze pad or cotton wool, should be left to heal. Water must not get in. Later if there is surface infection gentle cleaning and treatment with topical antibiotics and steroids, or boric acid powder, may be successful. Much rarer causes of continuing discharge are residual disease or metaplasia of the mastoid lining to one secreting mucus. Treatment of deafness after an ear is safe depends on the state of the other ear. The options are to do nothing, to offer a hearing aid, or to perform reconstructive surgery (tympanoplasty).

DEAFNESS IN ADULTS

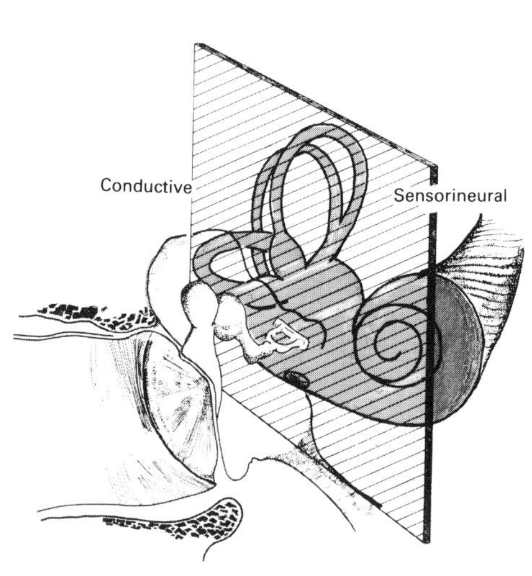

The effects of hearing impairment depend on the severity of loss, the rate of onset, whether one or both ears are affected, and the age of onset. A baby born deaf in both ears cannot learn to speak without special help, and normal language development will be impossible if the deafness is severe. A child with good speech will almost certainly lose it if severely deafened in the first years of life. An adult who becomes very deaf does not lose his or her vocabulary, but the lack of auditory feedback degrades the voice into a harsh flat monotone. Rapid total deafness in both ears is a catastrophe that affects every aspect of the victim's life, while gradually developing loss causes serious but less severe handicap. By comparison, total loss of hearing in one ear is relatively trivial, regardless of age.

Deafness is the cruellest form of sensory deprivation. Unlike blindness, it often provokes ridicule rather than sympathy. Unable to hear what is said and unable to control his own voice, the severely deaf person appears stupid. Isolated from family and friends and greeted by unsympathetic attitudes, he or she is often depressed. Tinnitus, which often accompanies deafness and is rarely found without it, can cause distress almost as great as that from lack of hearing.

The prevalence of hearing loss is not accurately known: probably over 3 million adults (6 in every 100 in the UK) have impaired hearing, and over 10 000 children need special education.

The two main types of defect are conductive and sensorineural. Conductive deafness arises from any impediment to the transmission of sound waves through the external ear canal and middle ear, as far as the footplate of the stapes. Sensorineural deafness implies a defect central to the oval window: in the cochlea (sensory), the cochlear nerve (neural), or, more rarely, in central neural pathways.

Conductive deafness

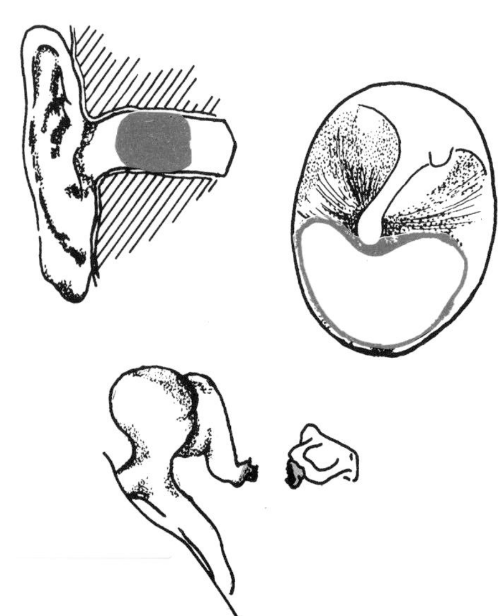

In conductive deafness there are five possible mechanical defects: (*a*) obstruction of the external ear canal; (*b*) perforation of the ear drum; (*c*) discontinuity of the ossicular chain; (*d*) fixation of the ossicular chain; (*e*) inadequacy of the Eustachian tube.

Obstruction—The external ear canal is most commonly obstructed by wax, but also by inflammation of the meatal wall and accumulation of discharge in otitis externa. Less common causes are congenital abnormalities of development (atresia), and foreign bodies.

Perforation of the ear drum impairs the transmission of sound by offering a reduced area for incident sound waves; by allowing sound pressure to be exerted adversely on the inner side of the membrane; and by exposing the round window membrane to incident sound pressure, which counters the normal route of transmission within the cochlea. Perforations usually result from infective damage but also from trauma, especially blows to the ear with the flat of the hand, and, more rarely, after sudden pressure changes during diving.

Discontinuity of the ossicular chain is usually a sequel to infective middle ear damage. The long process of the incus is most often destroyed. Injuries to the head or ear may dislocate one ossicle from another.

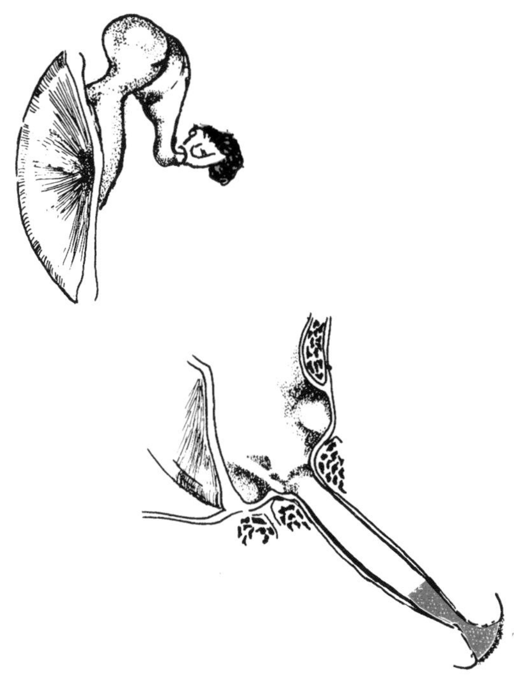

Fixation of the ossicular chain is the characteristic feature of otosclerosis. This inherited disorder fixes the footplate of the stapes in the oval window. No other part of the ossicular chain is affected. Otosclerosis must not be confused with tympanosclerosis, in which hyaline material is deposited under the mucosa of any part of the middle ear cleft, after repeated episodes of inflammation. These deposits may often be seen as "chalk patches" in the ear drum and they may restrict movement in any part of the chain.

Inadequacy of the Eustachian tube is common in children and is accompanied by accumulation of extremely viscous material in the middle ear—so called glue ear. Air is absorbed from the middle ear cleft; the tympanic membrane is pushed inwards by outside air pressure and its free vibration impaired; fluid then accumulates within the middle ear. Glue ear is the commonest cause of acquired deafness in children of school age. Apart from faults in the maturation of the normal tube opening, the nasopharyngeal orifice of the tube may be obstructed. The role of enlarged and repeatedly infected adenoids in preventing ventilation of the middle ear is controversial. Effusions in the adult middle ear are usually thin and serous. Although they often follow upper respiratory tract viral infections or barotrauma during aircraft descent, *carcinoma of the nasopharynx must be excluded* since it may present with a conductive deafness due to a middle ear effusion.

Sensorineural deafness

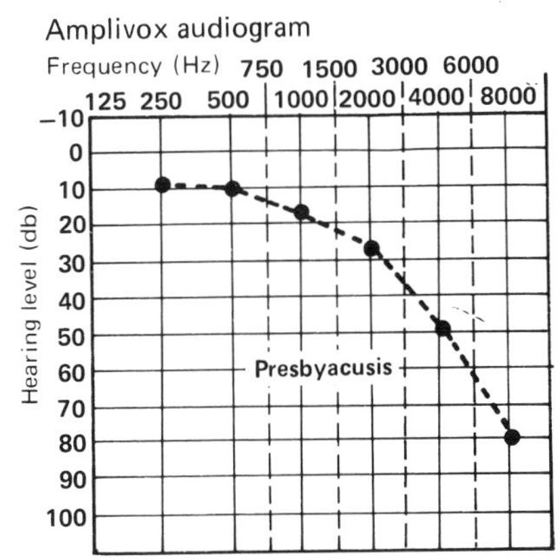

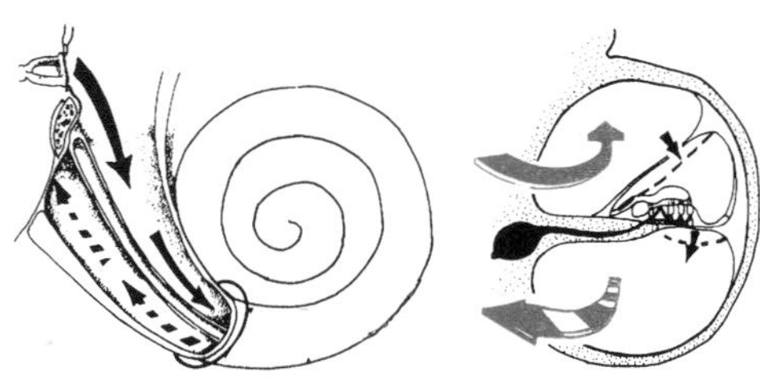

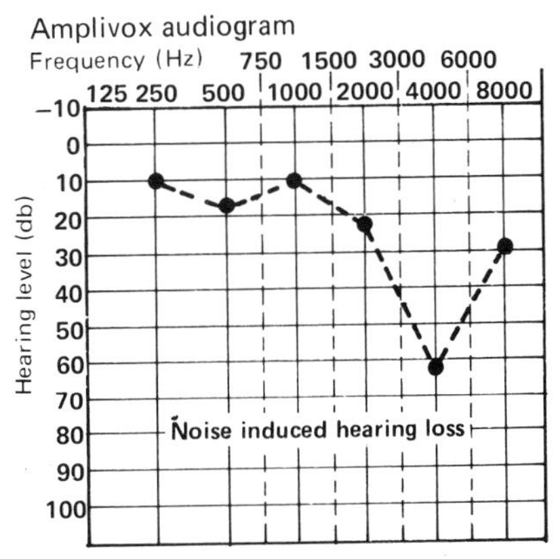

The three main patterns of sensorineural deafness are: bilateral and progressive, unilateral and progressive, and sudden.

The commonest reason for bilateral progressive sensorineural deafness is degeneration because of age—presbyacusis. A similar progressive hearing loss is sometimes seen in middle age as "presenile" degenerative change. Bilateral progressive hearing loss may also be caused by noise and by ototoxic drugs. Excessive noise damages the hair cells of the organ of Corti; the damage may follow brief high intensity exposure (acoustic trauma) but is usually caused by high intensity exposure over long periods. Such noise induced hearing loss is important in industry and is a hazard of noisy hobbies such as shooting and using power tools. The severity of damage depends on the intensity of the noise, duration of exposure, and individual susceptibility.

Ototoxic drugs—notably the aminoglycoside antibiotics—also destroy cochlear hair cells. Theoretically these antibiotics constitute a risk only when administered systemically, but topical applications—for example, of neomycin to large raw areas of body surface or to the bronchial tree as insufflations—are dangerous. Risks are greater in the elderly, those with impaired renal function, and after previous or concomitant ototoxic drug administration. Damage is irreversible and may continue after treatment has stopped. Blood concentrations before and after administration must be monitored. Some common diuretics—frusemide, when given intravenously, and ethacrynic acid—may be ototoxic. The well known ototoxic effect of large doses of salicylates is usually reversible.

When deafness is unilateral and progressive, Menière's disease (endolymphatic hydrops) or an acoustic neuroma must be considered.

Sensorineural deafness with a sudden onset is fortunately usually unilateral. One cause is trauma to the head or ear; if there is a leak of perilymph from the oval or round window membranes this may be surgically corrected. Other causes include viral infections (particularly mumps, measles, and varicella zoster) or sudden impairment of cochlear blood flow. Sudden hearing loss may also announce the presence of an acoustic neuroma.

Syphilis must always be considered with any pattern of acquired sensorineural hearing loss. In the past few years increasing numbers of cases of labyrinthine syphilis have been recognised. Serological investigations are essential whenever a reasonable explanation for the loss is lacking.

ASSESSING DEAFNESS

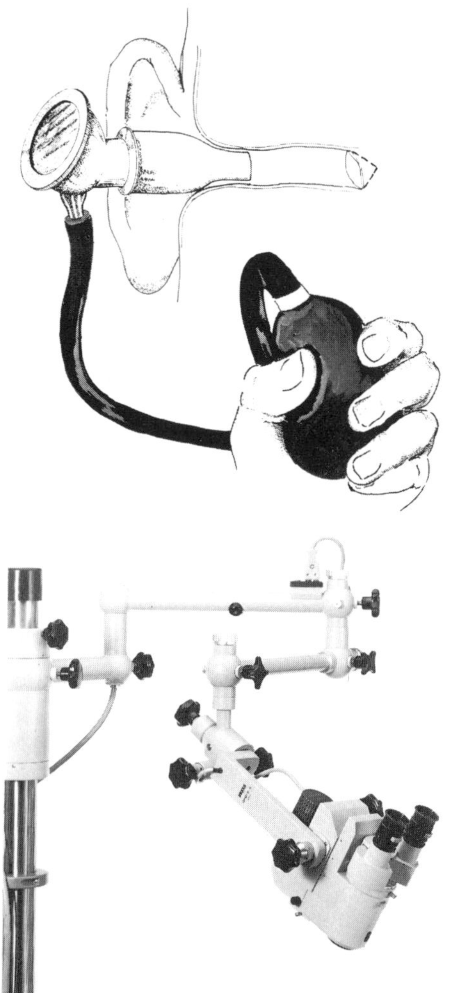

Full assessment of hearing impairment demands specifying, for each ear, the site of the defect, the cause, and the severity of disability and handicap. When these can be stated, which is not always possible, an attempt can then be made to determine (*a*) whether the defect is treatable, with a possibility of improving hearing; (*b*) the overall handicap, considering hearing in both ears, and (*c*) whether the deafness is a symptom of another disease—for example, syphilis or acoustic neuroma.

Important aspects of the history include the rate of onset and progression, family history, any information about noise exposure or unusual medication and associated aural symptoms (pain, discharge, vertigo, and tinnitus). Examination will show whether the external ear canal is obstructed and, if not, the state of the ear drum. Obstructing wax or debris must be removed. The otologist generally removes it manually under the illumination of a headlight using wax hooks and rings, or cotton wool on wire carriers, but the general practitioner may prefer to syringe wax from the ear. For safety there should be no previous history of middle ear disease or suspicion of perforation. A story of previous uneventful syringing is always comforting. If the wax is hard it may be softened by instilling olive oil or 5% sodium bicarbonate drops twice a day for a few days beforehand. Proprietary ceruminolytic drops should be used with great care since they may cause otitis externa with swelling of the meatal skin and severe pain if the canal is already filled with hard wax.

When the canal is clear the drum can be examined—preferably with a Siegle's speculum to assess mobility. Without this manoeuvre a middle ear effusion may be overlooked because the drum may look surprisingly normal when the whole middle ear is filled with mucoid material. At this stage the otologist will examine the ear under a binocular operating microscope.

Conductive and sensorineural hearing loss can be distinguished by the use of two tuning fork tests—the Rinne and the Weber. For each the ideal fork has a frequency of 512 Hz (cycles per second).

Rinne test

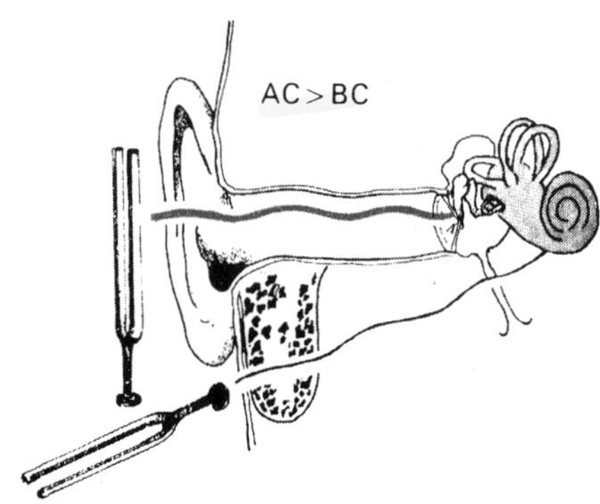

The examiner first establishes that the vibrating fork is audible at the meatus and on the mastoid process. The foot of the vibrating fork is then pressed on the mastoid bone of the ear under test. Then it is moved to the external meatus and the patient is asked whether he or she can still hear it. The fork is returned to the mastoid and the question repeated. By alternating this manoeuvre the examiner can establish reliably where the fork is heard longer. When conductive mechanisms are normal (giving a positive response, recorded as AC>BC) the test shows better (more prolonged) hearing by air conduction—at the meatus. Positive responses are found in normal ears, as would be expected teleologically, and those with sensorineural hearing loss.

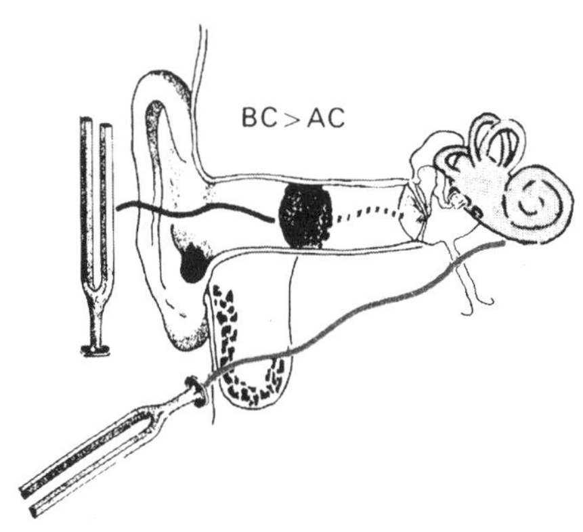

When the deafness is conductive, bone conduction, where sound is transmitted direct to the cochlea through the skull, remains unimpaired, while the response to sound conducted by air is diminished. As the hearing loss increases the sound is heard for longer by bone conduction than by air conduction. This is a negative response (BC>AC). If, however, one ear is totally deaf while the other retains good hearing, bone conducted sound from the deaf side will be heard by the intact cochlea on the other side, giving a *false negative Rinne* response. To expose this false negative the test should be conducted with a loud sound introduced into the normal ear—for example, with a Barany noise box.

A quicker way to carry out this test is to present the fork first by air conduction at the meatus, and then by bone conduction on the mastoid process, and to ask which stimulus seems louder.

Weber test

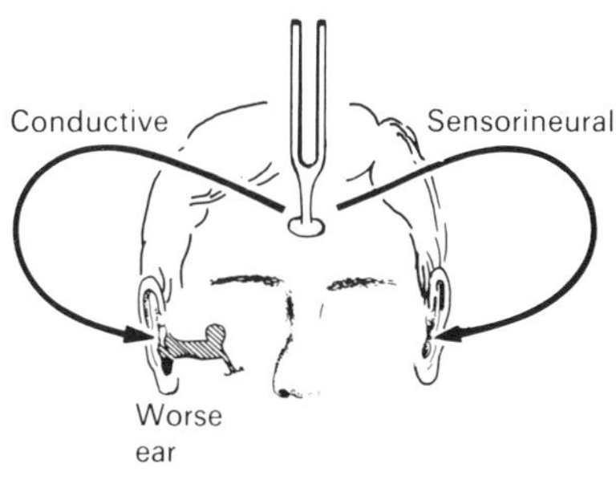

The foot of the vibrating fork is placed on the forehead and the patient asked in which ear the sound is heard. This test is particularly useful when hearing is very different in the two ears. When the hearing defect is sensorineural the fork will be lateralised to the better side. The reverse obtains when the deafness is conductive.

If there is a combination of conductive and sensorineural loss the normally reliable results of the tuning fork tests may be misleading.

Audiometric tests

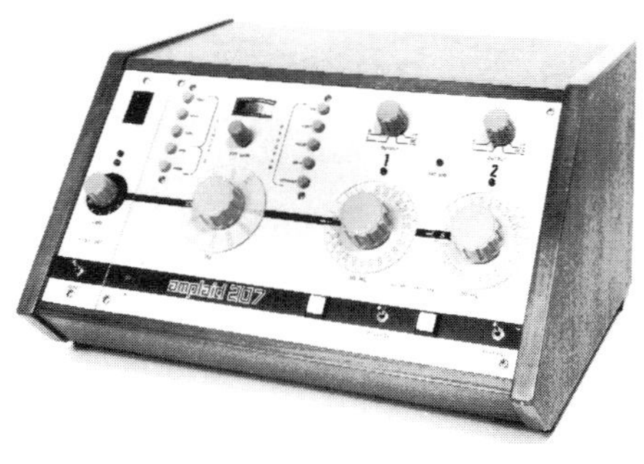

Amplivox audiogram

Frequency (Hz) 125 250 500 750 1000 1500 2000 3000 4000 6000 8000

Hearing level (db) −10 0 10 20 30 40 50 60 70 80 90 100

Conductive loss

[BC

●-● AC

Quantitative measures of the loss, and accurate determination of its site and cause, depend on audiometric tests.

The most familiar test is *pure tone threshold audiometry*. Performed with electronic equipment and standardised techniques in a soundproofed room this establishes the severity of the hearing loss throughout a range of frequencies from 250 to 8000 Hz. At each frequency the hearing loss is measured and plotted on a logarithmic decibel scale with reference to normal hearing at that frequency, to produce an air conduction audiogram. A bone conduction threshold audiogram can be produced by a transducer on the mastoid. By comparing the air and bone conduction thresholds a quantified Rinne test at different frequencies is available, allowing conductive and sensorineural hearing losses to be distinguished. Bone conduction thresholds must be regarded with caution. They are less accurate and reliable than air conduction thresholds.

A pure tone audiogram provides evidence of the type of hearing loss and indicates its severity. In some cases the pattern of the curve suggests the cause—for example, in hearing loss induced by noise, early Menières disease, and presbyacusis. More specialised tests in the outpatient clinic are needed to assess further the severity of the disability (though pure tone audiograms are surprisingly useful for this) but mainly to identify the site of the lesion.

Acoustic impedance measurements allow middle ear pressure to be assessed by *tympanometry* and middle ear effusions (otitis media with effusion) to be recognised. This technique records contraction of the stapedius muscle in response to auditory stimuli and is useful for recognising conductive defects and in sensorineural diagnosis.

Speech audiometry examines discrimination ability above threshold. It measures the proportion of spoken words recognisable at different intensities and, by comparison with the pure tone audiogram, indicates whether a sensorineural defect lies in the cochlea or auditory nerve. Tests for so called "loudness recruitment" and adaptation are also useful for distinguishing between sensory and neural defects. *Brain stem electric response audiometry* is now the technique of choice for making this distinction. This is the standard audiometric test used when an acoustic neuroma is suspected; it has high specificity and sensitivity. Final diagnosis now entails enhanced magnetic resonance imaging.

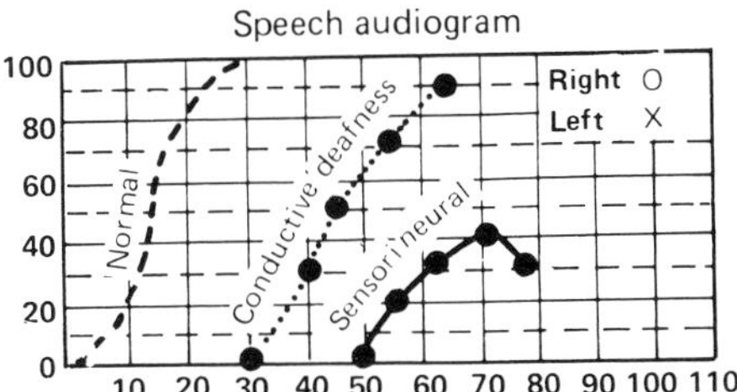

Management

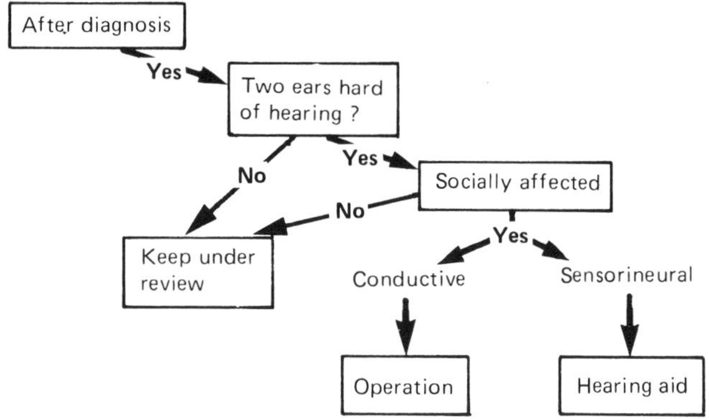

Apart from treating underlying disease, management must take account of the patient's social handicap (see next chapter). What can be done to help one ear depends on the state of the other. Theoretically most conductive defects can be remedied, while (with few exceptions) no correction is available for a sensorineural one. Apart from removing wax from the external meatus, conductive defects can be corrected by operations using the binocular microscope.

Surgery

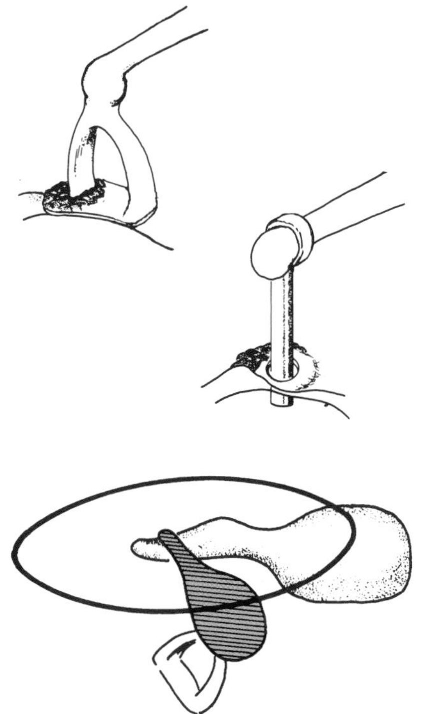

Stapedectomy—to correct otosclerosis—has led the development of microsurgery of the ear. The disability caused by the immobile stapes footplate is relieved by replacing the stapes with a plastic (or metal) prosthesis attached laterally to the long process of the incus and transmitting pressure medially to the perilymph of the inner ear within the vestibule.

Perforated ear drums are repaired by *myringoplasty*. A graft, usually of connective tissue (such as temporalis fascia), is placed usually on the inner surface of the drum after it has been prepared by removing the outer layer of skin.

Breaks in the ossicular chain are mended by various reconstructions (ossiculoplasties) to attach the ossicles to each other, using artificial materials such as hydroxyl apatite or ossicular bone. Rebuilding of both the ossicular chain and the defective drum is a *tympanoplasty*. (This term also describes reconstructive procedures in which diseased tissue is excised.)

Secretory otitis media (otitis media with effusion), particularly glue ear, is relieved by a myringotomy incision in the anterior ear drum, aspiration of the effusion (which is often difficult because of its tenacity), and insertion of a ventilation tube or grommet to ventilate the middle ear cleft.

All operations on the ear carry a risk of cochlear damage, particularly when the inner ear has to be opened as in stapedectomy. This risk determines the principle of operating on a patient's worse ear and never operating if a patient can hear with only one ear.

If neither surgery nor medical treatment can improve hearing, as in sensorineural deafness, the patient may need sound amplification with a hearing aid (see next chapter).

Sudden sensorineural deafness

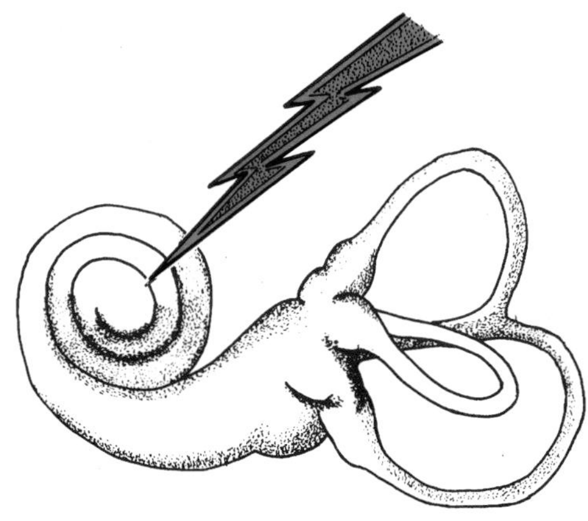

Sudden sensorineural deafness, which usually affects only one ear, constitutes a medical emergency. In most cases no cause is found. Fortunately the patient usually recovers or improves spontaneously after a few weeks. Nevertheless, all patients presenting with this syndrome should undergo full otological assessment. Some acoustic neuromas present in this way, as may syphilis. Traumatic tears of the intralabyrinthine membranes, with perilymph leakage from the oval or round window, may be preceded by the trauma of such slight exertion that it may escape the history. When this is possible the patient should rest sitting up in bed, and operative exploration of the middle ear may be considered to seal any perilymph leak.

If no cause is found and no perilymph fistula suspected treatment with systemic steroids and vasodilator drugs may be considered.

HELP FOR DEAF ADULTS

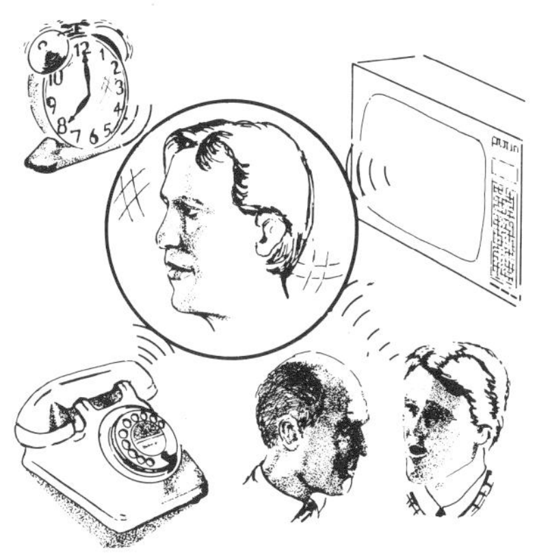

If more than slight, hearing impairment holds serious implications for the patient's family, social, and working life. Difficulties with a job may be exacerbated by the need to use a telephone. These generate financial worries, which, together with the problems of shared activities such as watching television or going to the theatre, create tensions in the home. The deaf patient becomes isolated and threatened and, not surprisingly, depressed. A major source of help is to provide a hearing aid.

Getting a hearing aid

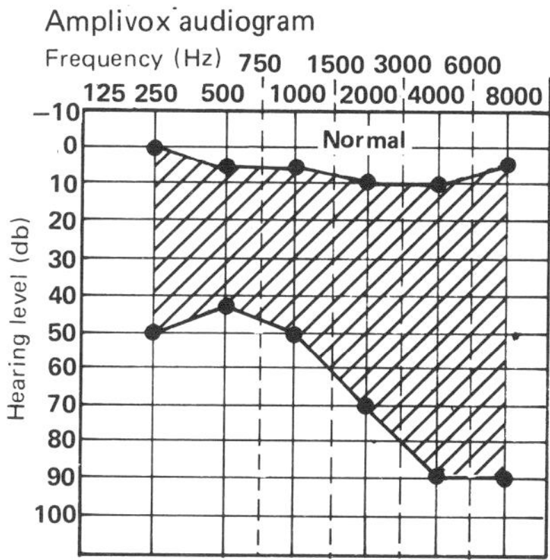

As a rough guide anyone whose pure tone audiogram in the better ear shows an average loss of 40 dB or more in speech frequencies (500, 1000, and 2000 Hz) is likely to have sufficient conversational difficulty to justify trial of a hearing aid.

Various hearing aids, both body worn and behind the ear, covering most needs are available through the NHS. The general practitioner should refer patients to the otolaryngology department of a hospital with facilities for distributing hearing aids. They will be assessed in the outpatient department before being fitted with an aid.

Alternatively, any patient may seek advice directly from a hearing aid dispenser. Their controlling body, the Hearing Aid Council, keeps a register of dispensers. If a hearing aid dispenser discovers that a patient might have conductive deafness or features other than those of a slowly progressive bilateral sensorineural loss the patient must, by law, be referred to the general practitioner. Many commercial dispensers will let a patient have an aid on trial for a time before purchase, and they have to make clear the terms of the trial. Patients should take advantage of such trials.

Types of hearing aid

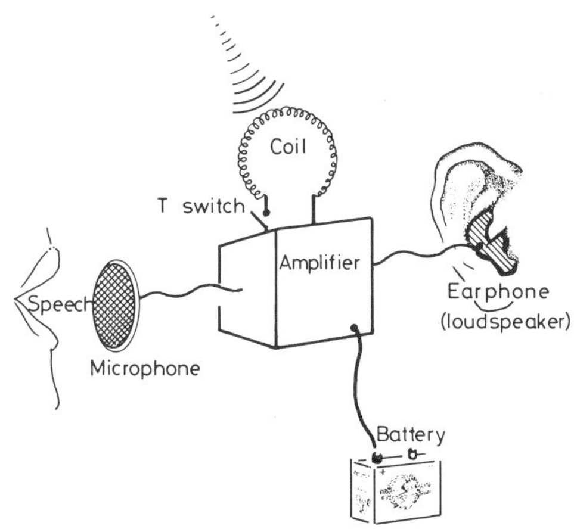

All electronic aids consist of a microphone, an amplifier, and an earphone. They are powered by dry batteries and have on–off and loudness controls. Some aids offer an induction coil or a T setting, which enables the aid to use electromagnetic induction fields and provides better quality sound from electromagnetic sources such as telephones, televisions, and microphones.

With some aids the amplifier and microphone are worn in a box on the chest with a wire attached to the earphone; in others all the components are in one small package on or near the ear. The latter, which are the more common, usually lie behind the ear with the microphone connected to the earphone by a transparent hollow tube. Some commercial aids incorporate the components in spectacle frames or increasingly in an "all in the ear" package.

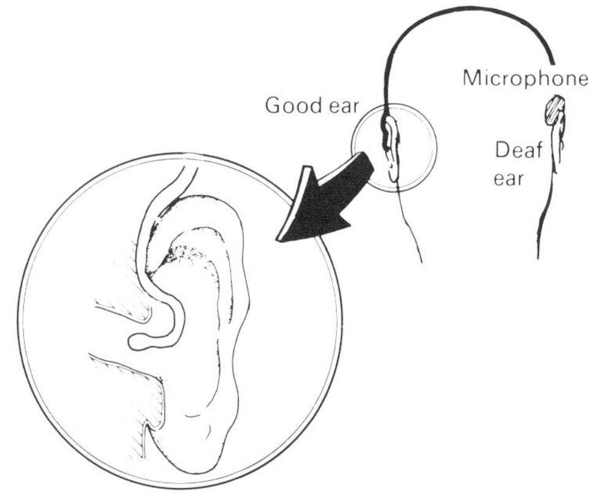

Aids differ electronically in terms of the gain, maximum output, and frequency response, and in measures to reduce the effects of sudden loud noise. They also differ in the way that sound is conveyed. This is usually to an insert which fits tightly into the meatus on the same side as the aid. This provides air conducted sound. Alternatively, sound may be conveyed to a bone conducting transducer pressing on the skull behind the ear. Sound may be taken from one side of the head to the other by a CROS (contralateral routing of signals) fitting. Two aids may be fitted, and combinations of transmissions from one side to the other provide varieties of CROS fittings.

Choice of aid

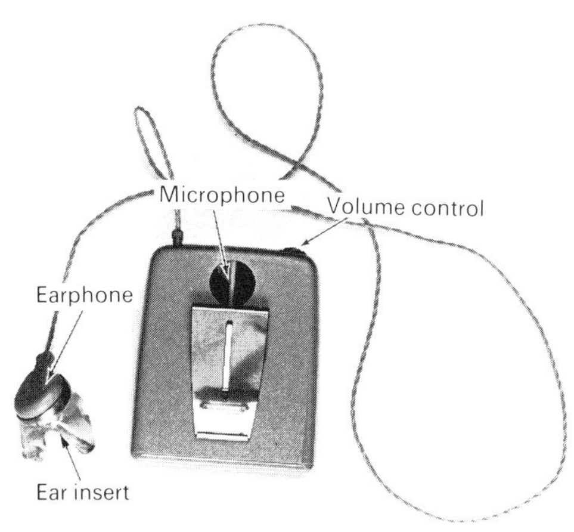

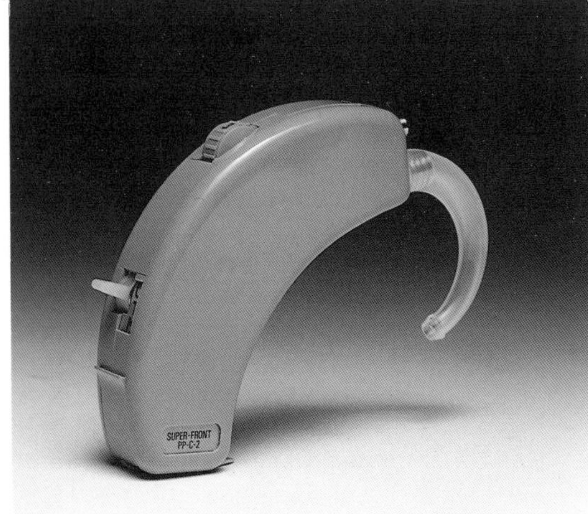

For an aid to be useful for speech discrimination the patient needs to distinguish at least half of speech content. Accurate prescription in the way that refractive errors are corrected is impossible. Even so, the unaided speech audiogram, and the presence or absence of recruitment (the phenomenon found with cochlear defects in which loud sounds are abnormally loud and often intolerable), will indicate the characteristics on which to base a choice for "trial and error."

An ear level, behind the ear aid, with a firmly fitting insert of hard acrylic, is the basic form of aid; it has various electronic features to suit most patients. A patient who is sensitive to loud noise will need some form of "automatic gain control" to reduce the effect of sudden loud noise. If very high amplification is needed there may be problems with acoustic feedback, producing the familiar high pitched whistling sound. This occurs whenever the outlet to the ear is not acoustically isolated from the microphone and will affect any aid with an insert that does not fit the ear tightly enough.

High gain that causes feedback despite a properly fitting insert demands that the microphone of the aid be separate from the earpiece. A body worn aid may be advisable. Alternatively, the aid can be connected by a CROS fitting. Body worn aids, apart from being conspicuous, cause unwanted noise from rubbing against clothes; ear level]af12aids may be affected by wind noise.

Some moulds cause allergic reactions in the external ear canal and alternative materials must be used. Any condition with discharge from the ear—a mastoid cavity, chronic middle ear disease, otitis externa—will be adversely affected by an airtight plug. One solution is to fit a bone conducting aid, but this needs greater power and causes discomfort because of the pressure needed to hold it to the head (by a springy headband or special spectacle frame). Another is an open mould, in which just the tip of a tube fits into the ear but does not occlude it, or a CROS fitting, with the aid on the other side to prevent feedback.

Arthritic patients may find the tiny controls of ear level aids hard to manipulate. Spectacle aids have the disadvantage that repair or loss of either spectacles or hearing aid deprives the user of both. Some commercial aids are now available with small remote control handsets to alter settings.

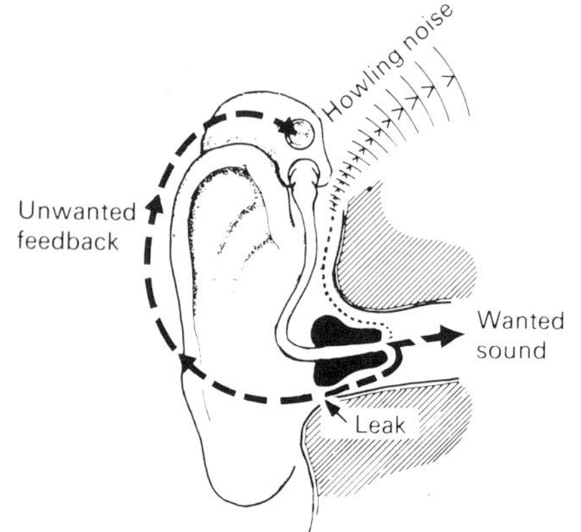

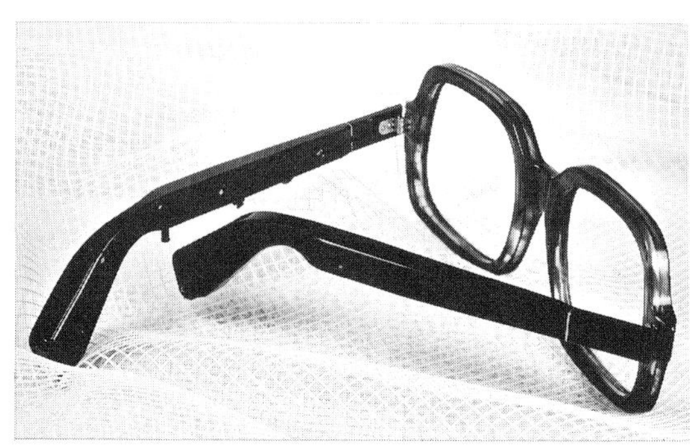

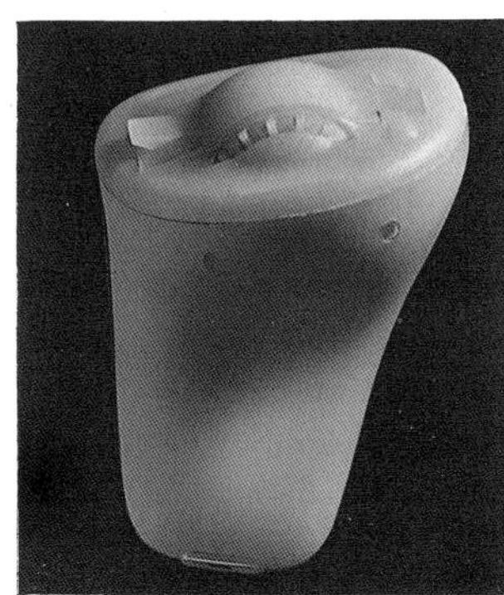

Which ear to fit?

- Fit better ear if neither is adequate unaided
- Fit poorer ear if better is useful without aid

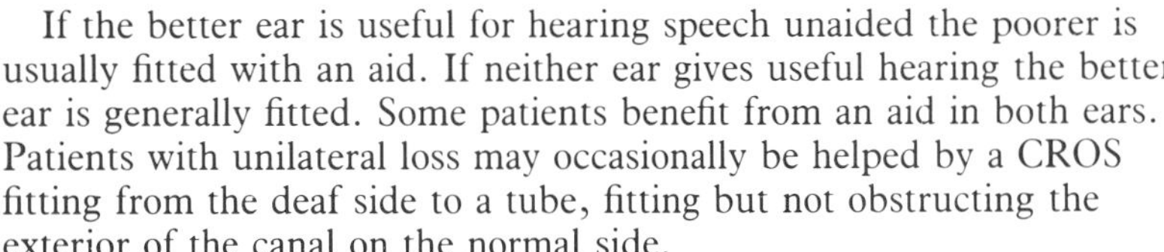

If the better ear is useful for hearing speech unaided the poorer is usually fitted with an aid. If neither ear gives useful hearing the better ear is generally fitted. Some patients benefit from an aid in both ears. Patients with unilateral loss may occasionally be helped by a CROS fitting from the deaf side to a tube, fitting but not obstructing the exterior of the canal on the normal side.

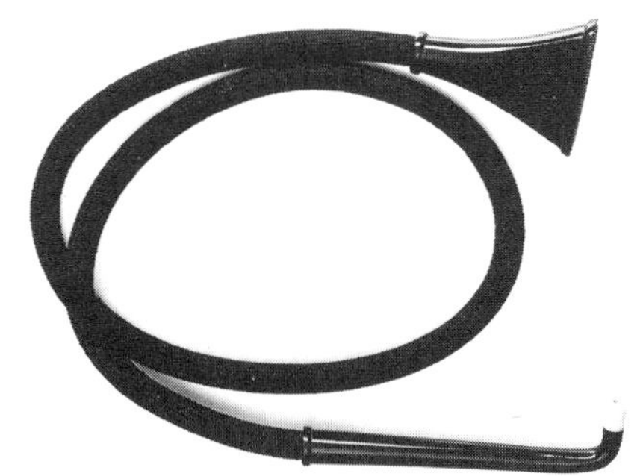

Even if an aid does not discriminate speech usefully it may help lip reading, indicating rhythms and cadences of speech; in the worst case it may be useful as a warning of impending danger.

It is a sad irony that hearing aids give best results for patients with conductive deafness, for whom there are often operative alternatives.

A patient may be disappointed once the aid is fitted if he or she expected nearly normal hearing. No aid provides normal sound, and patients need counselling and auditory training if their aids are not to end life in a drawer. They need to be encouraged and taught to interpret and use the sounds, distorted compared with normal hearing, that the aid can provide.

Old fashioned speaking tubes or ear trumpets may be surprisingly helpful for the very deaf.

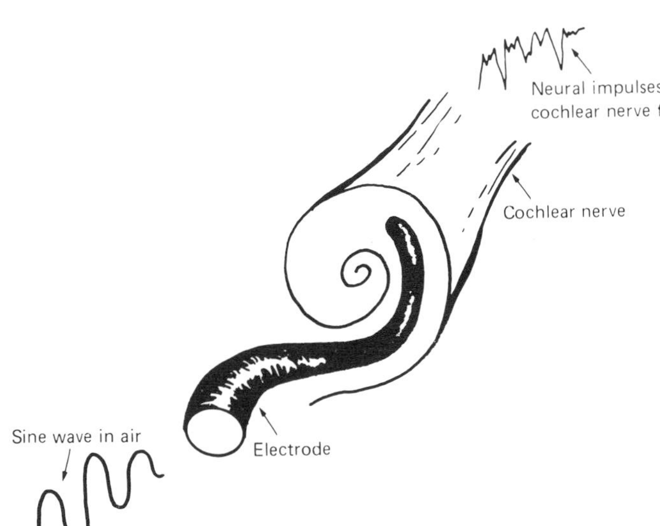

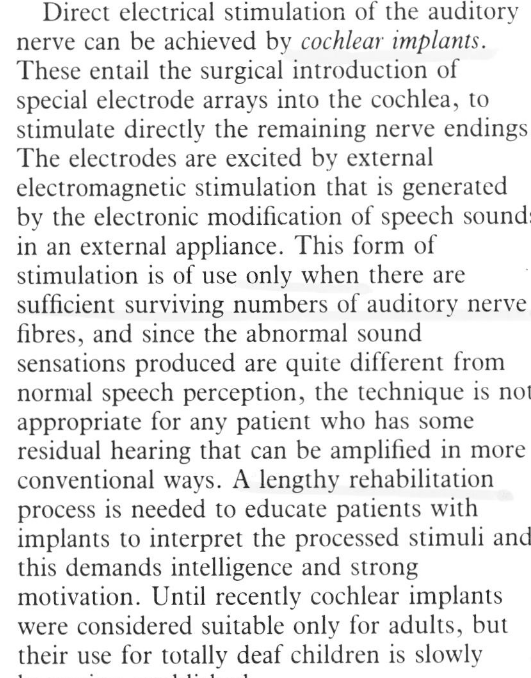

Direct electrical stimulation of the auditory nerve can be achieved by *cochlear implants*. These entail the surgical introduction of special electrode arrays into the cochlea, to stimulate directly the remaining nerve endings. The electrodes are excited by external electromagnetic stimulation that is generated by the electronic modification of speech sounds in an external appliance. This form of stimulation is of use only when there are sufficient surviving numbers of auditory nerve fibres, and since the abnormal sound sensations produced are quite different from normal speech perception, the technique is not appropriate for any patient who has some residual hearing that can be amplified in more conventional ways. A lengthy rehabilitation process is needed to educate patients with implants to interpret the processed stimuli and this demands intelligence and strong motivation. Until recently cochlear implants were considered suitable only for adults, but their use for totally deaf children is slowly becoming established.

Lip reading

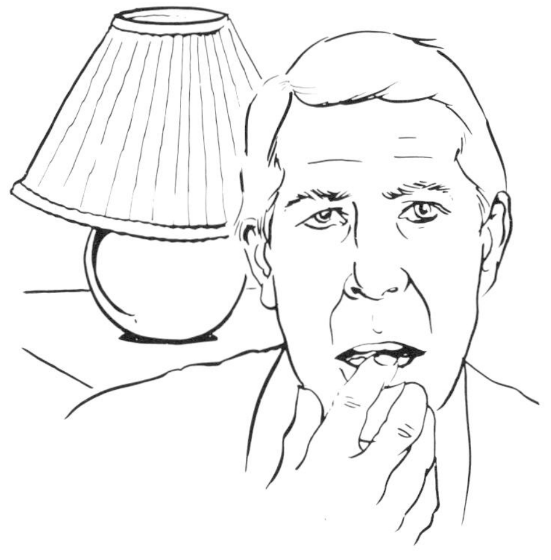

To be understood:
Do not obscure face
Do not sit in shade

All normally hearing people watch faces as a supplement to hearing, and instruction in lip reading is essential for any severely deaf patient. If a patient has a progressive hearing loss that will eventually become severe or total, help with lip reading should be sought while the level of hearing is still useful. The availability of instruction in lip reading varies. Advice should be sought from local adult education bodies, or, as with any problem raised by this chapter, from the Royal National Institute for the Deaf, 106 Gower Street, London WC1. In London the City Lit Centre for the Deaf provides advice and training in all aspects of auditory rehabilitation, lip reading, manual communication, and speech and machine shorthand (palantype) operation. The City Lit also runs a course for hearing therapists.

The effect of sudden severe or total deafness on a previously hearing adult is as apocalyptic as a major stroke. Patients and their families need help from psychiatrists, social workers, and teachers of the deaf. Ideally patients should have a period of residential care. They must never be left to fend for themselves in a silent world.

Link, the British Centre for Deafened People, at Eastbourne, is a registered charity providing residential rehabilitation courses, primarily for adults of working age who become the victims of sudden deafness.

Environmental aids

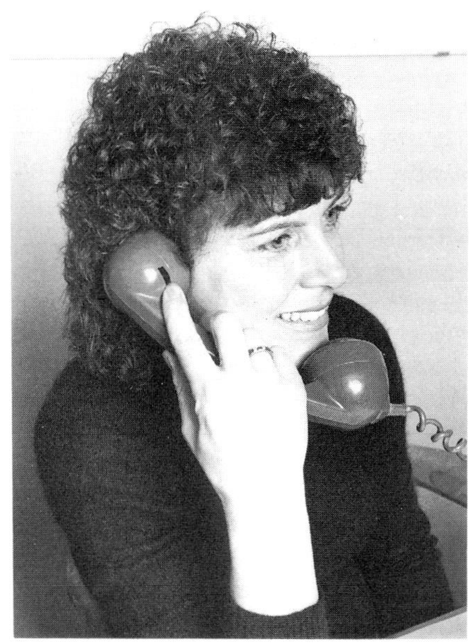

There are many fairly cheap aids that can make life easier for the deaf.

Telephones—Advice and devices are available from telephone sales offices: (*a*) bells may be replaced with extension bells, buzzers, hooters, or flashing lamps; (*b*) amplifying handsets provide an adjustable volume control; (*c*) inductive couplers provide an electromagnetic field which can excite an induction coil in a hearing aid in the T (telephone) position; (*d*) separate receivers allow a person with normal hearing to hear the call and "lip speak" to a deaf listener.

Watching television is socially less disruptive if the deaf patient can adjust his volume independently of the loudspeaker volume of the set. Most television retail or rental firms supply various devices. Television adapters have an isolating transformer that is attached to the set and linked by a wire to a gain control box to which the patient's earphone is connected. Induction loops are wires placed around a room from isolating transformers which generate electromagnetic fields that can be picked up by the induction coil of a hearing aid set in the T position. This provides better quality sound without interference from the amplification of unwanted environmental noise. Microphone aids, attached to the patient's ear through an amplifier, are stuck directly to the grill of the TV set.

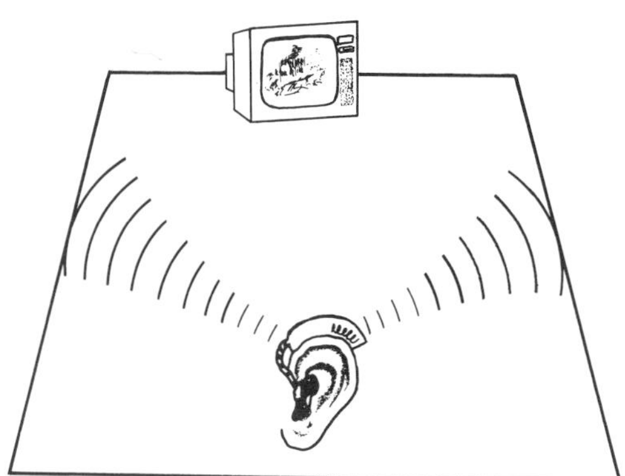

Teletext decoders allow the viewer to receive written information on his screen from Ceefax (BBC1) and Oracle (ITV). The user can select the information he or she wants. Oracle offers information on deaf societies as well as instruction in lip reading. A "mix" facility allows text to be shown over the programme on the set, which will be particularly useful when subtitles are more generally available. Prestel, which funnels information from telephone lines to the television set, offers much more information but not specifically for the deaf.

Alarms—Door bells can be modified to buzzers, lights, hooters or gongs. Baby alarms and clock alarms can also activate vibrators or lights.

Tinnitus

Sound perception from:

generation in environment

generation in body

Abnormal electrical activity = tinnitus

Abnormal brain = hallucination

For many severely deaf patients tinnitus is almost as worrying as the deafness. For some with moderate hearing loss tinnitus may be the dominating problem, while in a few a hearing defect is found only when tinnitus is investigated.

Very rarely tinnitus may be objective—that is, created by sound waves generated within the body by vascular tumours, abnormal blood flow, palatal myoclonus, or an insect in the meatus. The noise is then audible to an examiner. In conductive deafness tinnitus is often the effect of removing ambient masking noise so that body activities become audible.

Tinnitus in sensorineural deafness can be explained by a change in resting activity in the auditory nerve or its central pathways. Everyone experiences tinnitus at times and almost all will hear "white noise" when placed in surroundings which have been sound proofed. The resting magnitude of spontaneous activity in the auditory system is only just below that at which a sound enters consciousness: this is the price paid for the sensitivity of normal hearing. It is not surprising therefore that many mechanisms in sensorineural deafness may—for example, by affecting inhibitory influences on the cochlea—change the magnitude of resting activity and produce tinnitus. Perhaps it is also not surprising that there is yet no proved drug remedy for this symptom of protean inner ear malfunction. Carbamazepine is often worth trying, and the effects of local anaesthetics are under investigation.

Management of tinnitus

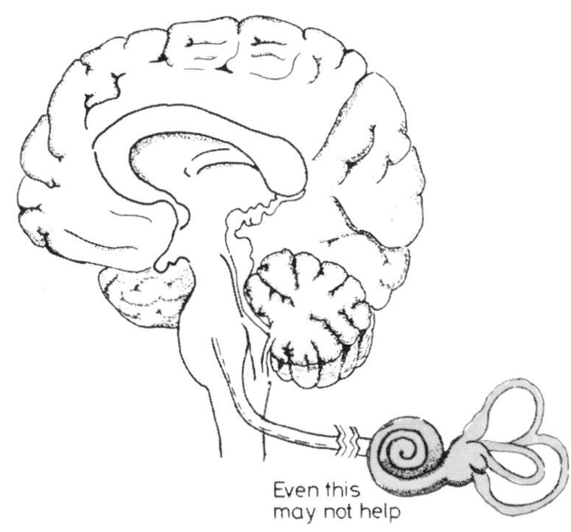

Reassurance—Many patients fear that tinnitus is a symptom of serious brain disease or impending stroke. Careful explanation of the mechanisms is time well spent.

Psychotherapy—There is a relation between tinnitus and depression, whereby the patient may blame the depression on the tinnitus, when in fact the relation is complex and two way. If depression can be identified and relieved tinnitus becomes much less troublesome.

Masking sound—Many patients find ambient noise helpful. At night this can be provided by the white noise of a radio tuned "off station." Tinnitus maskers, which look like hearing aids and produce different types of noise, are sometimes useful. They can be obtained on the National Health Service (subject to the resources of the otolaryngology department) and are available commercially. Their value can be assessed only by trial and error; for a few it is considerable.

Cochlear nerve section has only limited scope and should be considered only when an ear is totally deaf, since this measure produces relief in only about half the patients. Tinnitus can be worse afterwards so the possibilities and risks must be discussed carefully with a psychologically stable patient.

DEAFNESS IN CHILDHOOD

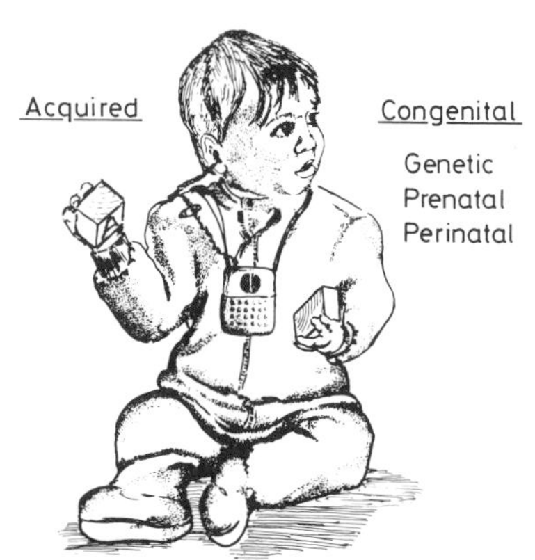

Without hearing a child cannot acquire language, nor can he develop normal relationships. One to two of every 1000 liveborn infants suffer from deafness. Childhood deafness may be congenital or acquired. Congenital deafness may be (*a*) *genetic*, due to inherited defects; (*b*) *prenatal*, due to events during pregnancy such as rubella, cytomegalovirus or other virus infections, or the effects of drugs such as thalidomide that cross the placental barrier; or (*c*) *perinatal*, due to events at or around the time of birth. These include birth trauma, anoxia, and haemolytic disease of the newborn with kernicterus.

Deafness in the first few years of life may be due to virus infections such as measles or mumps, meningitis, ototoxic antibiotics, or other causes already discussed in relation to adults.

Screening

The aim should be to recognise every deaf child by the age of 8 months to 1 year—before the vital time for learning speech is wasted. Any medical or surgical causes need treatment, and training in acquisition of language should be started as soon as possible.

Certain high risk groups may be recognised. They are likely to be seen in paediatric clinics, from where they will be referred, if thought to be deaf, to the audiology clinic. At risk are those with a family history of deafness, those born after maternal problems in pregnancy, those with perinatal problems, those with cerebral palsy or meningitis, and those whose speech is delayed or faulty. Any child whose mother believes her child to be deaf should also be suspect. Mothers are rarely wrong in this suspicion.

Screening of these high risk children will nevertheless overlook more than one third of deaf children and, ideally, screening should comprise examination of all infants in the population at child health clinics. Hearing *must* be assessed at 8 to 9 months and again on school entry. An additional assessment at 2 to 3 years is highly desirable. If deafness is suspected the infant is referred to an audiology centre for assessment by a senior clinical medical officer or a paediatric audiologist working with an educational audiologist or teacher of the deaf.

High risk groups

- Family history of deafness
- Maternal problems in pregnancy
- Perinatal problems
- Cerebral palsy
- Delayed or faulty speech

Screening methods

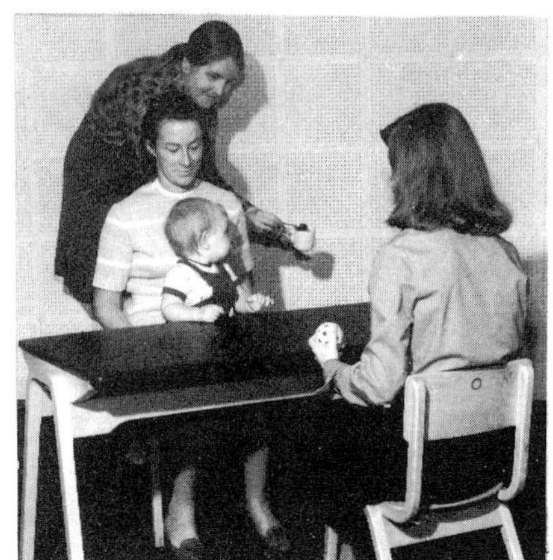

Screening methods depend on age. During the first 6 months there should be a "startle" or auropalpebral reflex in response to short bursts of high intensity sound. A mother's observations are very important. The startle test produces many false positive responses.

The second 6 months of life are the most important because hearing is easily testable and any loss discovered is early enough for help. At this age the normal child is sitting up and can be tested by distraction techniques. Appropriate sounds, presented at ear level about three feet away, cause a normal child to turn towards them. The sound must be meaningful to the child. Low frequencies can be produced by the spoken voice, high frequencies by a special rattle. Crinkled tissue paper provides a broad spectrum stimulus. These distraction techniques need two assessors—one to engage the child's attention (but not too much) and the other to make the noise. The assessor has to ensure that the response is to sound and not to movement seen or felt.

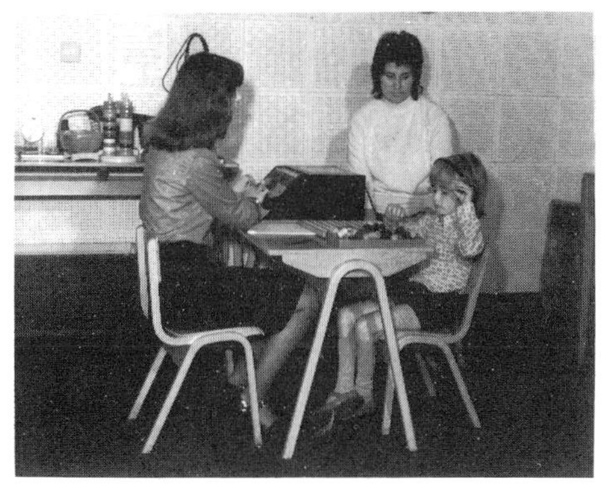

From 12 months to 2 years children become uncooperative and difficult to test. Quiet speech, with an expectation of comprehension, is an appropriate stimulus.

By the age of 3 children are once again cooperative but any severe hearing loss should have already been discovered. In addition to assessing speech comprehension, pure tone audiometry is possible using free field sounds, then an earphone can be held to the ear, and finally earphones may be fitted. The child is conditioned to react to the stimulus—for example, by putting a brick into a box when he hears the sound.

Audiometry, training, and aids

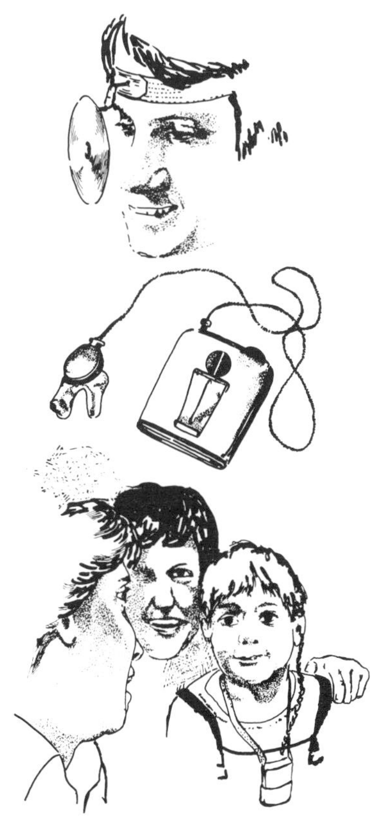

Techniques with electric response audiometry (including electrocochleography) and other measurable responses to sound stimuli are available in special clinics when simpler tests give equivocal results and accurate information is needed. Such assessment may be necessary if suspected hearing loss is associated with other disabilities. No child is too young or too difficult to test with these techniques.

At all times the possibility of surgical correction of conductive deafness, such as that produced by glue ear, must be kept under consideration. Acquired middle ear effusions, so common in childhood, may exacerbate existing sensorineural hearing loss and are more prevalent in babies than used to be thought.

Once deafness is diagnosed the child is referred to an otologist in an otolaryngology department for assessment of cause and possible treatment. Concurrently the teacher of the deaf plans auditory training and arranges the fitting of a hearing aid, and the child's progress will be regularly assessed in the audiology clinic. Between the ages of 2 and 3 years decisions about the child's future education are made. The goal is to achieve competence in language by the age of 5.

Auditory training involves exposing the child to normal speech sounds so that with the help of an aid residual hearing can be used in learning to discriminate speech differences and in monitoring the child's own attempts at imitation. Parents need to talk as much as possible to their child in a normal way.

Children usually need higher gain from their hearing aids than adults, and the fact that the child is growing produces difficulties in mould insertion and instrument management. Although very powerful aids are often needed there is no proof that they may damage residual hearing, though investigations are continuing.

Education

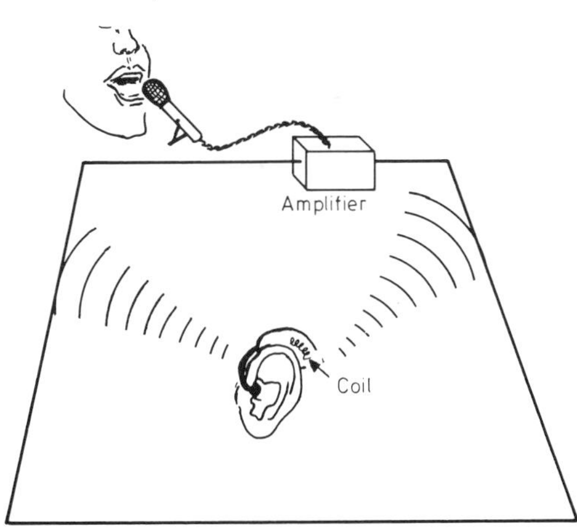

Deaf children may be educated in a normal school, in a partially hearing unit in a normal school, or in a school for the deaf. About half the deaf children attend normal schools, where they are seen by visiting teachers of the deaf. They advise on use of hearing aids, help with lip reading, and assess progress. A very deaf child has great difficulty in using a hearing aid with the background noise of a normal classroom.

Partially hearing units, which are increasing in number, offer the facilities of special classrooms, like those in schools for the deaf, within a normal school. Special schools for the deaf take about half the deaf children, usually from 3 to 18 years. Their classrooms are fitted with induction loops allowing the induction coil of the hearing aid to respond to the teacher's voice transmitted over a microphone while the child moves around. Better reception is gained from a radiomicrophone system, where the teacher speaks into a lightweight microphone and the sound transmitted is received by a radioreceiver worn by the child. Various arrangements take the received signal to the child's hearing aid.

The majority view in the United Kingdom favours an exclusively oral approach to education of deaf children

The consensus emphasis in education in the United Kingdom is on oral methods, whereby the development of language and speech is encouraged with the use of residual hearing and amplification by hearing aids. Alternative (manual) forms of communication have certain disadvantages, in particular the need for long and repeated practice and the possibility of using skills only with others similarly trained. Combinations of oral and manual methods are termed "total communication." Forms of manual communication include finger spelling—the traditional deaf and dumb alphabet; cued speech, in which the signs made near the mouth are used to resolve ambiguities in lip reading; and signing systems, such as the British and Paget–Gorman systems, in which signs indicate words, ideas, and grammatical distinctions.

Swimming with grommets

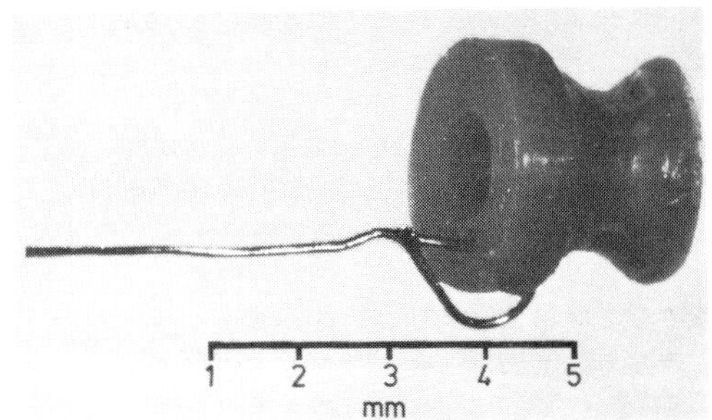

Swimming is always an important and controversial issue for children. With a grommet in place the ear should be protected against water. Swimming in swimming baths should ideally be banned because the chemical irritant of chlorinated water in the postnasal space is a potent predisposing factor in secretory otitis media and acute otitis media, even in ears without grommets.

A child with a grommet may bathe safely in the sea but parents should be warned not to allow submersion or diving. The drum can be protected during bathing with a large piece of cotton wool, moistened with petroleum jelly, in the external meatus. Fitted plugs to seal the meatus can be made by hearing aid dispensing firms and provide better protection for an ear with a grommet in place. A child with a grommet who develops otitis media will suffer less pain than one with an intact drum but discharge may be profuse. The usual treatment for otitis media with systemic antibiotics should be given and the ear mopped dry. Antibiotic and steroid drops may then be instilled.

Acquired conductive deafness

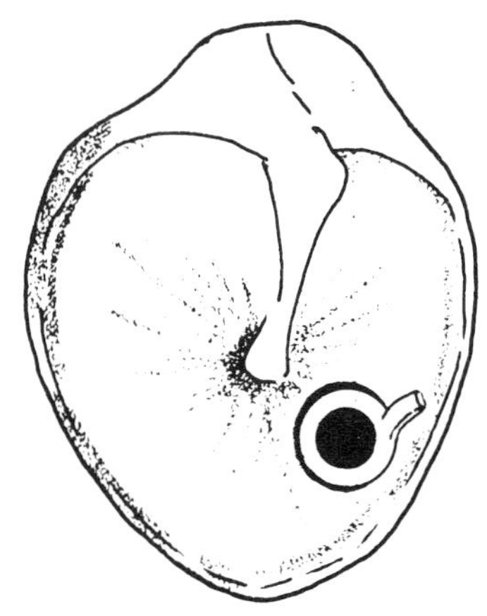

The commonest cause of acquired deafness in childhood is secretory otitis media (otitis media with effusion). When first discovered it is reasonable to wait four to six weeks in the hope that the effusion may resolve. During this time decongestion of the nasopharyngeal mucosa is useful and this may be encouraged by oral antihistamines together with decongestant nosedrops—1% ephedrine in normal saline or xylometazoline hydrochloride (Otrivine)—provided they are not used continuously for over two weeks. If the effusion persists operation will be needed. Myringotomy is performed under general anaesthesia, the effusion aspirated, and a grommet inserted through the myringotomy incision. The operation is often performed as a "day case." The grommet allows air into the middle ear, a role eventually assumed by the Eustachian tube.

A grommet will become blocked by wax and surface keratin on average about 6 to 9 months after insertion. Then it will be embedded in wax and gradually extruded along the external ear canal to the exterior. It will fall out or easily be removed with forceps.

Sometimes the condition recurs and repeat insertion of a grommet may be needed, occasionally up to five times. Long term grommets, such as T tubes, which can be expected to stay in place for two or three years, are often used after a second recurrence. Little can be done to prevent recurrence. The role of adenoidectomy is controversial but it may occasionally help.

VERTIGO

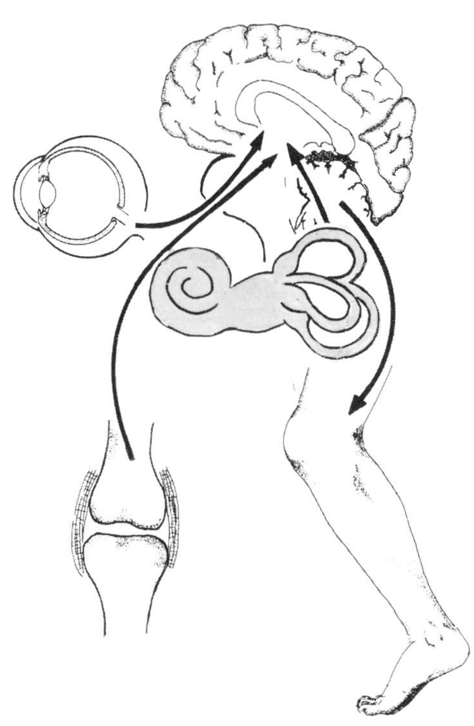

Vertigo is an illusion of movement, when a patient wrongly believes that he or the environment is moving. It is not a synonym for imbalance; vertigo is always associated with imbalance but imbalance is not always due to vertigo.

Correct balance requires (*a*) accurate sensory information from the eyes, proprioceptive receptors, and the vestibular labyrinth; (*b*) accurate coordination of this information within the brain; and (*c*) a functioning motor output from the central nervous system to a normal musculoskeletal system. A defect in any of these systems will impair balance.

Vertigo occurs when the information from vestibular sources conflicts with that from other sensory systems or when a disordered central integration system cannot coherently assess the body's movements from vestibular information. Vertigo is always a symptom of a vestibular defect. The defect may lie in the peripheral labyrinth or in its connections within the brain—the brain stem, the cerebellum or the temporal lobe cortex. When severe it is usually accompanied by nausea and vomiting.

Vertigo is caused by: (*a*) *peripheral vestibular* (*labyrinthine*) *disorders*; (*b*) *central vestibular disorders*, due to multiple sclerosis, tumours, infarcts, abscesses; and (*c*) *external influences on the vestibular system* including drugs, anaemia, hypoglycaemia, hypotension, viral infection, syphilis, and most important, because of its potential danger, erosion of the bony walls of the labyrinth by destructive middle ear disease with cholesteatoma.

The commonest peripheral vestibular disorders are Menière's disease and other forms of endolymphatic hydrops; benign paroxysmal positional vertigo; sudden vestibular failure; and vascular disturbances. These account for over 75% of cases of vertigo.

Menière's disease

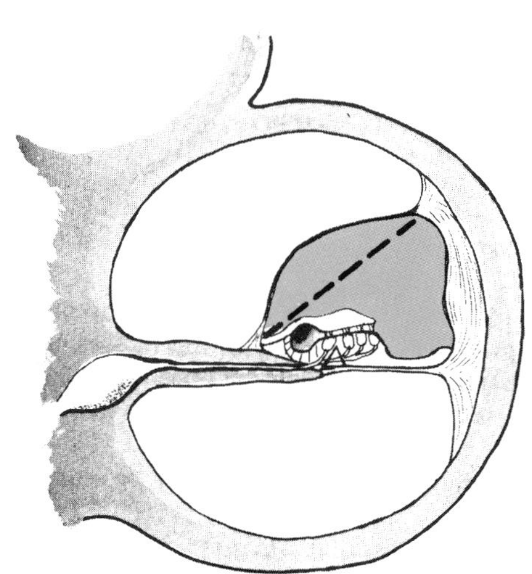

Menière's disease is a disorder of endolymph control characterised by dilatation of the endolymphatic spaces of the membranous labyrinth. Dilatation, or hydrops, may be caused by disorders of the otic capsule such as labyrinthine syphilis, or previous labyrinthine damage; but in Menière's disease the hydrops is idiopathic.

The disease usually affects only one ear and most often first produces symptoms between the ages of 30 and 60. It is characterised by attacks of violent paroxysmal vertigo, often rotatory, associated with deafness and tinnitus. Attacks usually occur in clusters, with periods of remission in between, when balance is normal. An attack lasts for several hours—rarely less than 10 minutes or more than 12 hours—and is generally accompanied by prostration, nausea, and vomiting. A sensation of pressure in the ear, an increase or change in the character of tinnitus, pain in the neck, or increased deafness often precedes an attack. Loss of consciousness is rare and suggests epilepsy.

The accompanying deafness is sensorineural and fluctuates in severity. It is associated with distortion of heard speech and musical sounds and with severe discomfort on exposure to loud noise. The fluctuating hearing loss may develop before the first attack of vertigo, although both symptoms often occur together. Even so, the deafness may not be noticed during the all consuming experience of vertigo. Hearing tends to improve during remissions, but over time it deteriorates, fluctuating until the loss becomes severe. The tinnitus is roaring or low pitched and worse when hearing is most impaired.

Menière's disease
- Paroxysmal vertigo
- Fluctuating sensorineural deafness
- Tinnitus

In the 20–30% of patients with bilateral Menière's disease deafness tends to become more serious than the vertigo. A form of *vestibular hydrops* produces attacks of Menière-like episodic vertigo, but without auditory symptoms. Another variant of Menière's disease is *cochlear hydrops*, which is a very common cause of fluctuating hearing loss, with tinnitus and distortion but without vertigo.

Benign paroxysmal positional vertigo

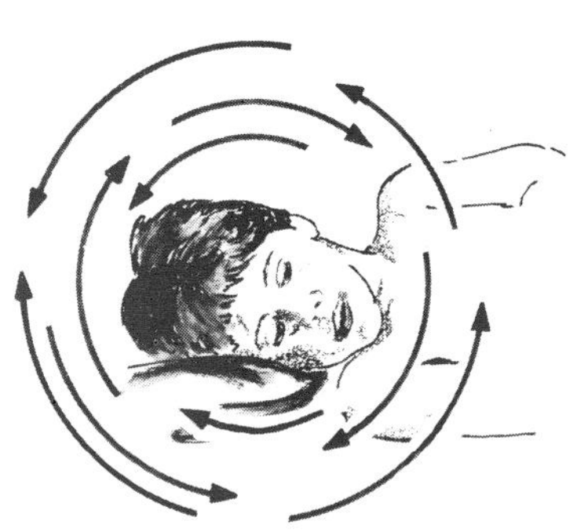

Benign paroxysmal positional vertigo is the commonest cause of vertigo. It is provoked by movements of the head, usually to one side when turning in bed or on looking upwards. Each attack lasts for only a few seconds, though it may seem longer to the patient, and there are no auditory symptoms.

The disorder is due to detachment of calcium carbonate crystals from the otoconia of the otolith organ of the affected utricle. These fall against the cupula of the posterior semicircular canal. The cause may be injury, viral infection, or degenerative changes with aging but often there is no explanation. Attacks are provoked only by adopting the specific position of the head and they usually stop after a few weeks or months, but they may recur.

Sudden vestibular failure

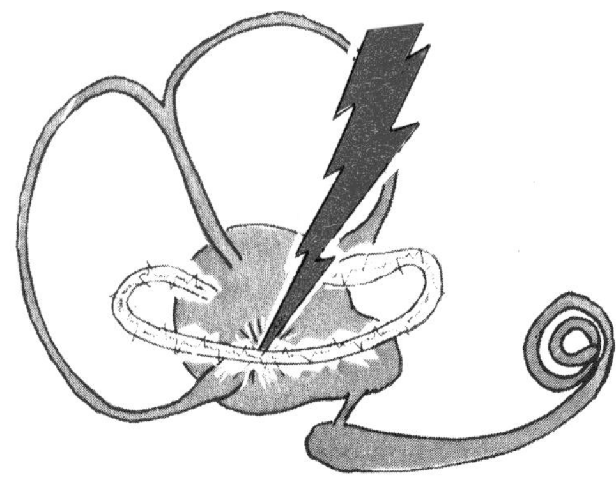

Sudden vestibular failure occurs when one peripheral labyrinth suddenly stops working. This may happen for various reasons, including closed head injuries, viral infection (such as by varicella zoster), blockage of an end artery supplying the labyrinth, multiple sclerosis, diabetic neuropathy, and brain stem encephalitis. The effects are sudden vertigo with prostration, nausea, and vomiting. There are no auditory symptoms, and the vertigo persists continuously, gradually improving over many days or weeks. Vertigo is exacerbated by head movements, but after a few days it may be absent unless the head is moved. The patient gradually regains his balance so that on the third or fourth day after onset he can move unsteadily around the room, holding on to furniture. By the end of 10 days he can usually walk without support if he avoids sudden movement. After three weeks gait may seem normal but the patient still feels insecure, particularly in the dark or when he is tired.

Recovery is slower and less complete in old age. It depends on compensating changes within the brain, and imbalance may return temporarily whenever the acquired compensation breaks down—for example, through defects in other sensory systems, fatigue, other illness, drugs, or the cerebral degeneration of old age.

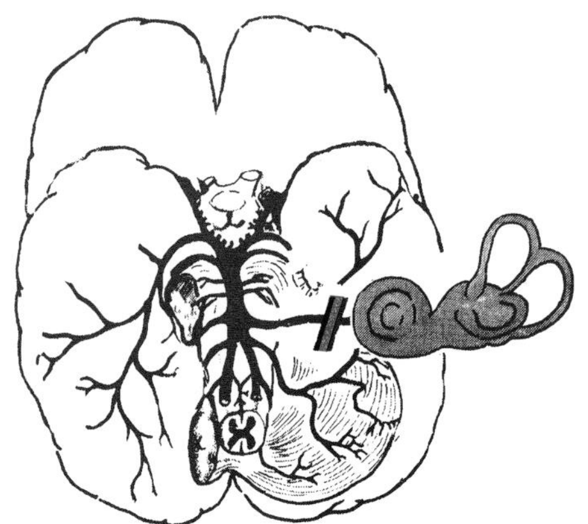

Migraine may cause episodic vertigo indistinguishable from that of Menière's disease.

Basilar migraine typically affects adolescent girls, causing symptoms similar to those of Menière's disease preceded by dimming or loss of vision due to ischaemia of the posterior cerebral artery territory. The vertigo is often associated with dysarthria and tingling in both hands and feet. Severe occipital headache may follow the attack.

Obstruction of an end artery supplying the labyrinth may produce the syndrome of vestibular failure.

Vertebrobasilar ischaemia is a central vascular disorder. Usually affecting older patients with degenerative vascular disease, it is characterised by attacks of vertigo associated with other symptoms of cerebral ischaemia such as dysphasia, paraesthesiae, weakness of the limbs, and visual disturbance.

Assessment and testing

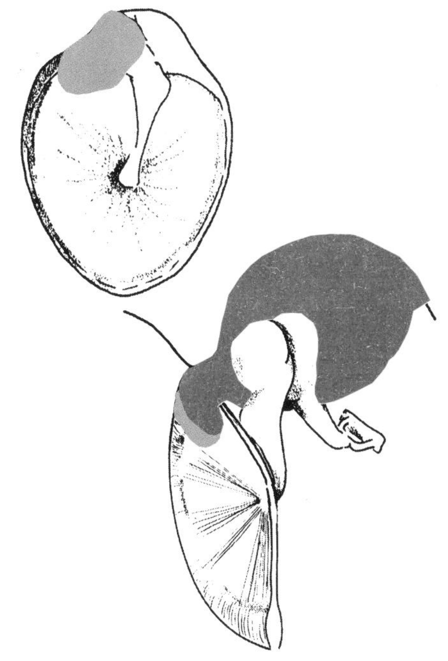

The doctor's first task is to recognise the symptom as vertigo and then to determine whether there is any systemic cause or extralabyrinthine disorder needing urgent investigation—destructive middle ear disease or any central vestibular abnormalities. The history is the doctor's most useful tool.

Clinical examination must include assessment of the cardiovascular and central nervous systems. Careful examination of the ears is the only way of recognising destructive middle ear disease with cholesteatoma. Suspicion must remain until each tympanic membrane is found to be normal. A wax crust over the pars flaccida is deceptive since it may cork the entrance to an attic cholesteatoma. If there is any doubt referral for examination under the microscope, which may require general anaesthesia, is essential.

Spontaneous jerk nystagmus is always a sign of vestibular disease. Its assessment requires examination of the eyes under good illumination. Inspection in all positions of gaze is necessary, but the eyes should not be abducted more than about 30°—until the edge of the iris reaches the caruncle. The following characteristics of a jerk nystagmus always indicate a central cause: (*a*) the nystagmus persists for more than a few weeks without abating; (*b*) it shows a change in the direction of beat (defined by the direction of quick component) either with time or change in direction of gaze; (*c*) it beats in any direction other than horizontally; (*d*) it is different in the two eyes (ataxic). Stance and gait should be examined by watching the patient standing with eyes closed and walking heel to toe.

Positional testing

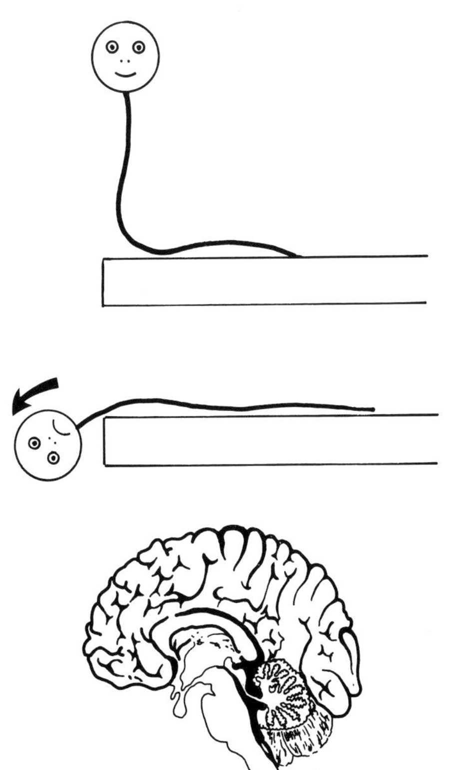

Simple positional testing is most important. Seated on a couch the patient turns his head towards the examiner and is told to keep his eyes on the examiner's forehead. The examiner, holding the patient's head, rapidly lays him back into a supine position with his head over the edge of the couch—30° below the horizontal. The examiner holds him there for at least 30 seconds, while watching the patient's eyes for nystagmus. The test is then repeated with the head turned to the other side. Nystagmus provoked by this test is always an abnormal finding.

Positional nystagmus is found in benign positional vertigo, but it can also, rarely, indicate a vestibular lesion somewhere in the posterior cranial fossa. In benign paroxysmal positional vertigo the nystagmus invariably shows the following features: (*a*) it is rotatory, beating towards the underlying ear; (*b*) a latent period of some seconds precedes its onset; (*c*) it abates after 5–20 seconds in the provoking position and is less violent on repeated testing; (*d*) it is accompanied by violent vertigo; (*e*) it does not change direction during observation. If any of these features is lacking a central cause must be sought.

Vertigo of central origin should be suspected (*a*) when there are other neurological symptoms such as visual disturbance, dysphasia, parasthesiae, or weakness of the limbs; (*b*) when the story does not fit into one of the peripheral labyrinthine patterns, in particular if the vertigo and vomiting are less conspicuous than continuing or deteriorating imbalance and ataxia; (*c*) when other neurological abnormalities can be shown; (*d*) when spontaneous jerk nystagmus has central features or positionally provoked nystagmus lacks the peripheral features described above.

Further tests

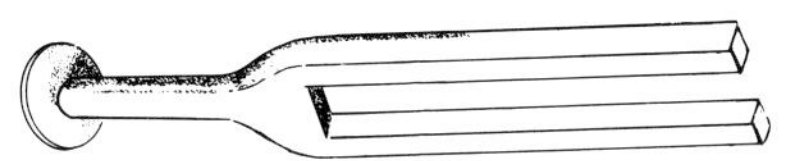

Examination next requires assessment of hearing, firstly with tuning fork tests to identify any sensorineural hearing loss. Further assessment demands referral for neuro-otological investigations of auditory and vestibular function.

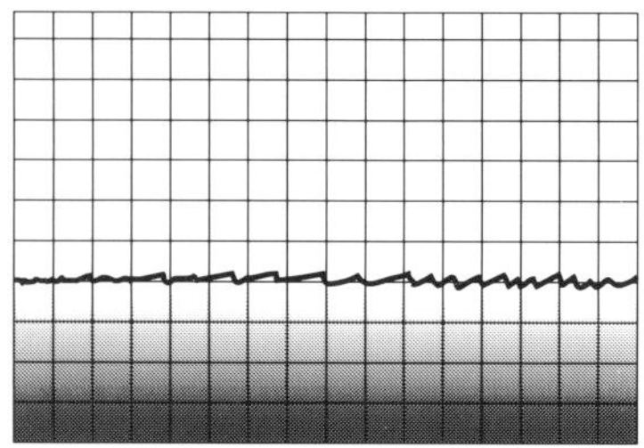

Electronystagmogram

In tests of vestibular function the labyrinth is vicariously stimulated by irrigation of the ears with water at temperatures other than body temperature (caloric tests), or by rotating the whole body at variable angular acceleration. The induced nystagmus may be observed for duration or recorded by electronystagmography (ENG), which allows measurement of such features as the speed of eye movements in a particular direction. ENG also gives valuable diagnostic information about spontaneous nystagmus.

Additional investigations should include serological tests for syphilis.

Symptomatic treatment

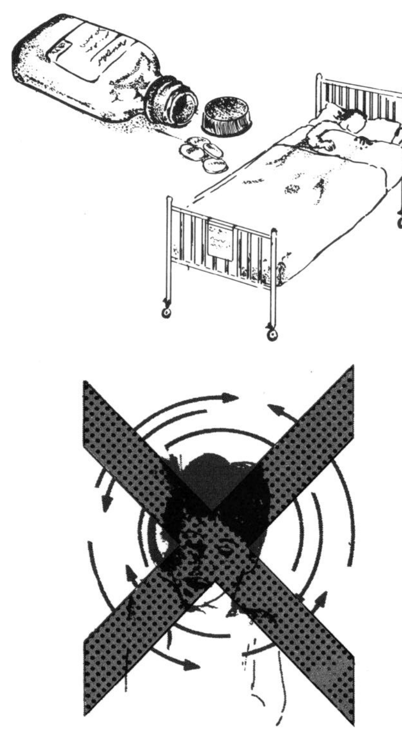

When conditions demanding referral for further investigation or treatment have been excluded, reassurance to explain that this cataclysmic symptom is not due to serious disease is important. Symptoms may be relieved by sedatives such as prochlorperazine, cinnarizine, and other antihistamines. Diazepam is also useful. If an attack is severe bedrest will be necessary whatever the cause of the vertigo. If vomiting prevents oral administration of drugs they may be given intramuscularly or as suppositories. Once the acute stage is over sedatives may be continued in small doses for several weeks or months.

If a vestibular deficit, rather than irritation of a more or less normal labyrinthine system, is pronounced vestibular sedatives may exacerbate the symptoms. This often occurs with the degenerative changes of old age; in bilateral Menière's disease and labyrinthine syphilis; or when the labyrinths have been severely damaged by ototoxic drugs. Patients can be helped by graded head and eye movement exercises, designed to accelerate the process of central compensation. These Cawthorne–Cooksey exercises are taught and supervised by physiotherapists. Exercises that cause vertigo may help adaptation in victims of benign positional vertigo, but these patients generally need only to avoid the provoking head position, while those with sudden vestibular failure need reassurance and symptomatic treatment.

Other forms of treatment are directed at recognised causes and include surgical exploration of any middle ear in which cholesteatomatous erosion of the middle ear is suspected. If a labyrinthine membrane rupture is suspected after trauma the middle ear may have to be explored to seal a possible perilymph fistula.

Treatment of Menière's disease

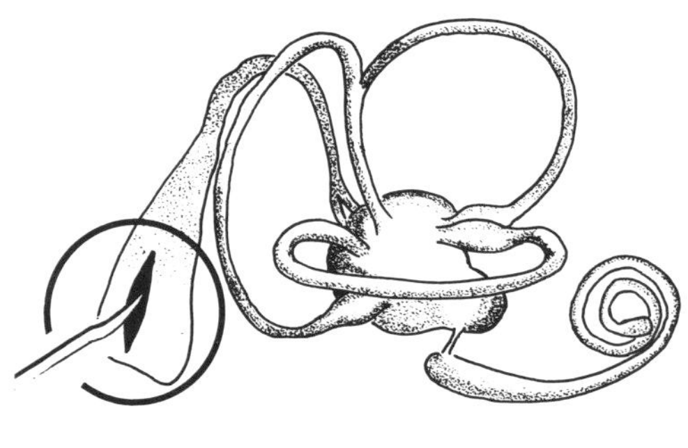

Medical treatment—There is some evidence that the endolymph disturbance has a vascular cause, and vasodilator drugs may be useful; betahistine hydrochloride 8 mg three times a day may be used if there are no contraindications such as a peptic ulcer. Nicotinic acid in a dose sufficient to cause flushing is an alternative. There is also evidence that Menière's disease might be due to electrolyte imbalance, and a salt restricted diet combined with a diuretic such as frusemide or hydrochlorthiazide may be useful.

Operation may be advised if the symptoms are not controlled by medication and reassurance. Conservative surgical procedures, such as *saccus endolymphaticus decompression operations*, aim to preserve hearing in the affected ear. These carry little risk of further auditory damage and are valuable in relieving attacks of vertigo; they may also prevent progress of the disease. Other conservative measures include selective division of the vestibular branch of the vestibulocochlear nerve (*vestibular neurectomy*). *Labyrinthectomy*, or total destruction of the membranous labyrinth, offers the most certain guarantee of relief from the vertigo of Menière's disease but at the expense of total loss of hearing in that ear. This is acceptable when hearing is already reduced to a distorted shred and the other ear retains normal function.

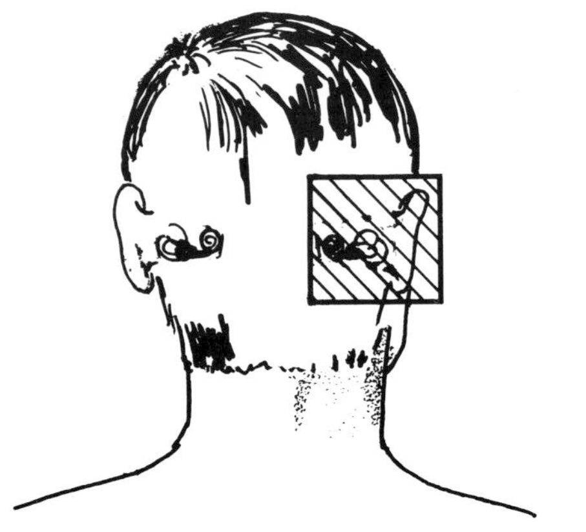

FACIAL PALSY

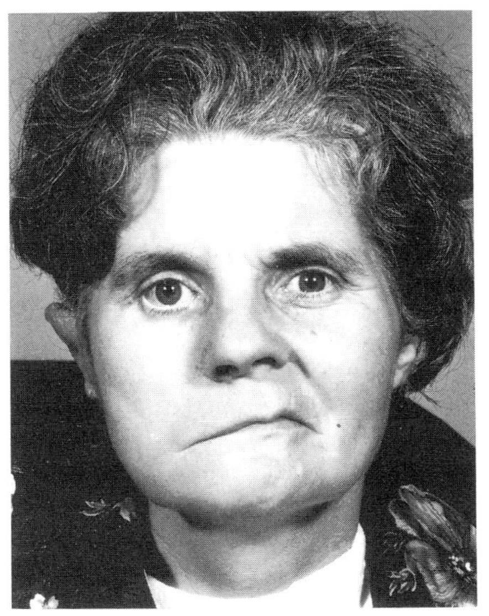

Two thirds or more of occurrences of lower motor neurone facial palsy are idiopathic. But idiopathic (or Bell's) palsy should be diagnosed only after a full investigation and after no other explanation can be found.

Intracranial causes of lower motor neurone facial palsy include neoplasia, multiple sclerosis, brain stem infarction, cerebellopontine angle lesions, and poliomyelitis. Intratemporal causes include trauma from an accident or surgery, otitis media (especially chronic with cholesteatoma), herpes zoster oticus (Ramsay Hunt syndrome), and carcinoma of the middle ear or neurofibroma of the facial nerve. The commonest extracranial causes are trauma and carcinoma of the parotid gland. Other causes include infectious mononucleosis, sarcoidosis, Lyme disease, severe hypertension—especially in childhood—and polyneuritis.

For a full diagnosis the doctor needs to identify the site of the lesion, its cause, and its severity.

Clinical assessment

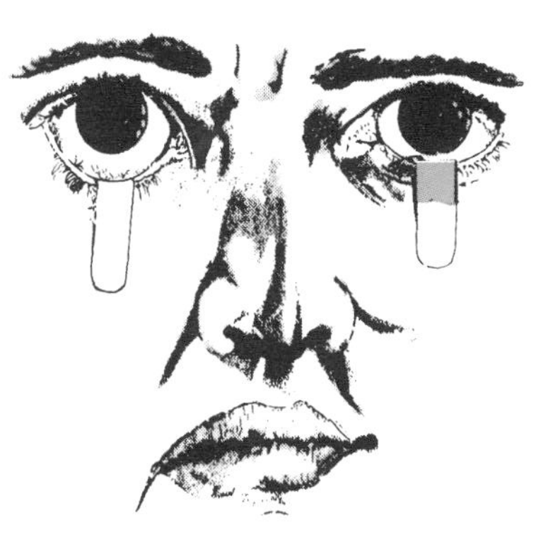

Recognising facial palsy depends on carefully examining the face during voluntary and involuntary (emotional) movement. The amount of weakness in the forehead, eyelids, nostrils, and mouth should be assessed. An unaffected forehead and paralysis on voluntary but not involuntary movement suggests an upper motor neurone lesion, which demands neurological examination.

The ear drums must be carefully examined. Cholesteatoma hidden by a crust over the outer attic wall is easily overlooked, but if it is suspected the patient must be referred urgently for surgical exploration. Chronic destructive middle ear disease should also be suspected if the patient has discharge, deafness, or symptoms of other complications such as vertigo. Inspection of the pinna and ear canal may show the rash and blisters typical of zoster infection in the Ramsay Hunt syndrome, in which paralysis and rash is preceded by pain.

Assessing the integrity of branches of the facial nerve requires examination of lacrimation and taste.

Lacrimation is easily tested by Schirmer's test. A folded strip of sterile filter paper is hung on the lower eyelids and the rate of lacrimation along each strip compared.

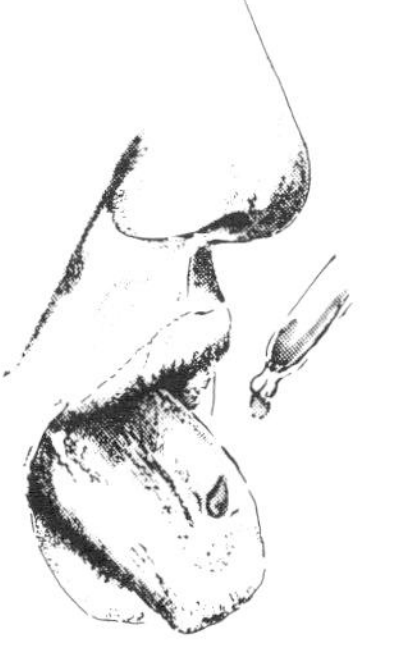

Taste on the anterior two thirds of the tongue is harder to test, and the patient's observations about disturbed taste at the time of onset of facial paralysis are often more useful than tests. The tongue should be dried with a swab and salt or sugar deposited on the anterior two thirds and the patient asked to comment.

Radiographs of the temporal bone are necessary if the cause of the palsy is not apparent. Computed tomography scans can be used to demonstrate the course of the nerve through the temporal bone and a role is developing for the use of magnetic resonance imaging.

Site of the lesion

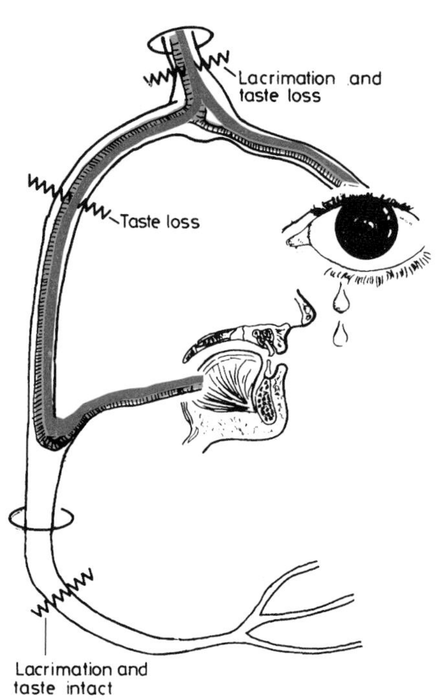

Branches of the facial nerve affected by paralysis will suggest the site of the lesion in the nerve. From the geniculate ganglion in the petrous temporal bone the great superficial petrosal nerve carries fibres to innervate the lacrimal gland. Just before it leaves the temporal bone (above the stylomastoid foramen) the facial nerve is joined by the chorda tympani, which carries sensory fibres from taste endings on the anterior two thirds of the tongue (plus secretory motor fibres for submandibular and anterior lingual salivary glands). Slightly above this a small branch supplies motor fibres to the stapedius muscle.

A lesion in the brain stem will produce only weakness of the facial muscle with no loss of taste or lacrimation. There are usually other neurological signs such as palsy of the VIth nerve, which causes diplopia due to weakness of the lateral rectus muscle.

Loss of lacrimation and taste from the anterior two thirds of the tongue suggests a lesion between the brain stem and geniculate ganglion.

Facial weakness with loss of taste but normal lacrimation indicates a lesion between the geniculate ganglion and the origin of the chorda tympani.

If both taste and lacrimation are preserved the lesion is peripheral to the stylomastoid foramen. There are no other cranial nerve defects and the lesion is usually obvious.

If the nerve has been affected by injury or disease this is usually apparent from the history or clinical examination—for example, aural discharge. In rare cases surgical exploration may be necessary to establish the diagnosis. In most cases, however, if the facial paralysis is of sudden onset and there is no apparent explanation on clinical or *x* ray examination, it is Bell's palsy. Some patients suffer several attacks of Bell's palsy.

Severity of lesion

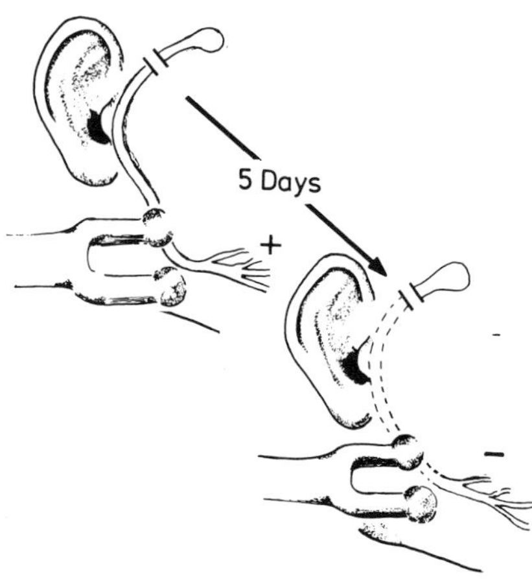

It is important to discover whether the nerve has suffered damage from which it will recover (neuropraxia) or more severe damage that will require regeneration for partial recovery (neuronotmesis or axonotmesis). Severity is usually assessed accurately by electrodiagnostic tests, but neuropraxia may be assumed unless one side of the face is completely paralysed.

If a nerve is suddenly damaged—for example by injury that divides it—no electrical test will show any abnormality until the peripheral part of the nerve has degenerated to the region where the test stimulus is applied. This distal degeneration will take from three to five days to reach the stylomastoid foramen, where nerve conduction tests are performed. Indeed, if the tests are normal one week after onset degeneration has not occurred even though the face may be completely paralysed.

Treatment

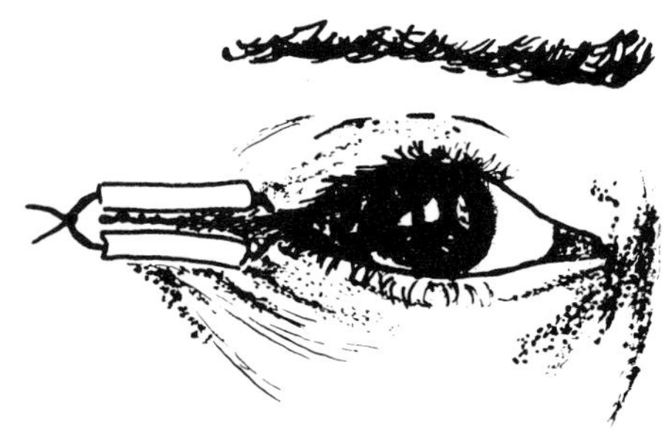

The aims of treatment of any facial palsy are to treat any lesion, alleviate the disability, and provide the nerve with the best chance of recovery.

The cornea of the eye on the affected side must be protected. An eye cover or spectacle wing may be adequate for a short period. But if recovery is expected to take months, a lateral partial tarsorrhaphy is advisable.

Facial appearance may be improved by lifting the corner of the mouth with a hook or filling out the cheek with a plumper, both of which can be attached to an upper denture. Massage or electrical stimulation of the paralysed muscle does not prevent atrophy or encourage recovery but it may boost the patient's morale.

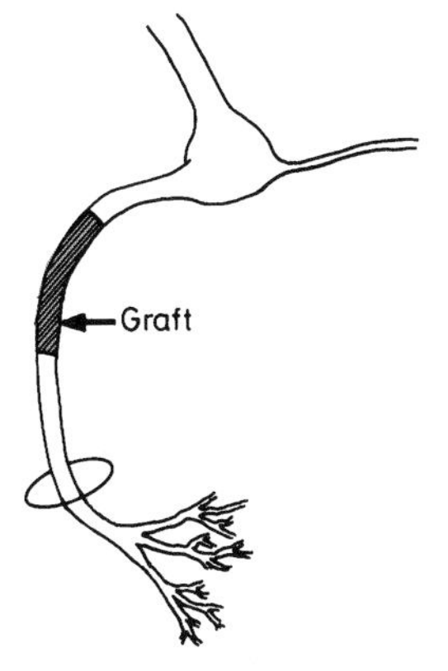

Help for the nerve depends on whether the fibres remain in continuity or whether they have been severed and their ends separated. If some voluntary movement remains, or if electrical responses remain normal for a long period, continuity is certain. If total degeneration is indicated by electrical tests and there is any doubt about the continuity, as after injury or chronic middle ear disease, surgical exploration is necessary to determine the state of the nerve. At operation breaches of continuity may be mended by rerouting the facial nerve within its temporal course or by inserting a "cable" nerve graft taken from the lateral cutaneous nerve of the thigh, the sural, or the great auricular nerve.

Treatment of Bell's palsy

Contraindications to steroids

Hypertension	Pulmonary tuberculosis
Pregnancy	Peptic ulcer
Diabetes	Middle ear infection

Bell's palsy is possibly due to ischaemia of the nerve within its bony canal. The value of systemic steroids is controversial but there is enough evidence in their favour to warrant their use when there are no contraindications such as hypertension, pregnancy, diabetes, pulmonary tuberculosis, peptic ulcer, or middle ear infection. Prednisolone 20 mg four times a day should be started as soon as possible after the onset of palsy, continued for five days, and tailed off gradually over a further five days.

If total degeneration has occurred in Bell's palsy there may be a case for surgical decompression to allow the oedematous contents within the sheath to swell without compression.

Prognosis

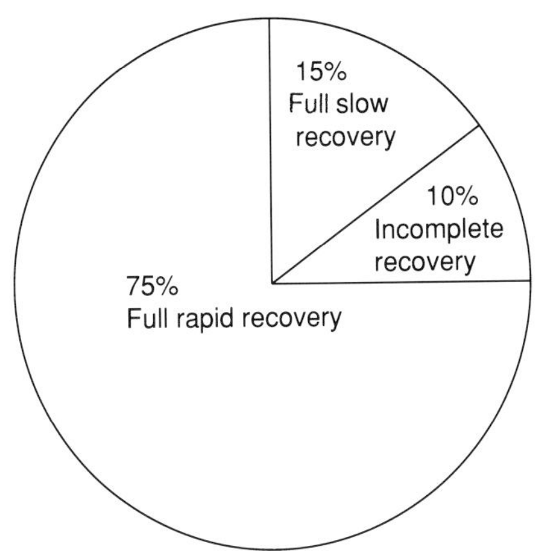

The prognosis depends on whether the nerve has degenerated. If there is no degeneration (neuropraxia) recovery is always complete, provided the cause is controlled. If there is degeneration recovery will depend on whether the nerve is in continuity. If it is, regeneration can occur, but it will take many months and the paralysis will recover only partially, with associated movements, contractures, and sometimes involuntary clonic spasm.

In Bell's palsy 90% of patients recover fully. Seventy five per cent suffer neuropraxia and can expect normal movement to return within three weeks of onset. Of the remainder (those who suffer degeneration) about half face the prospect of slow and incomplete recovery. The extent of neural damage is usually set at onset but a few patients experience further deterioration during the first week or so. Repeat attacks are less likely to resolve than initial ones.

Treatment of failed degeneration

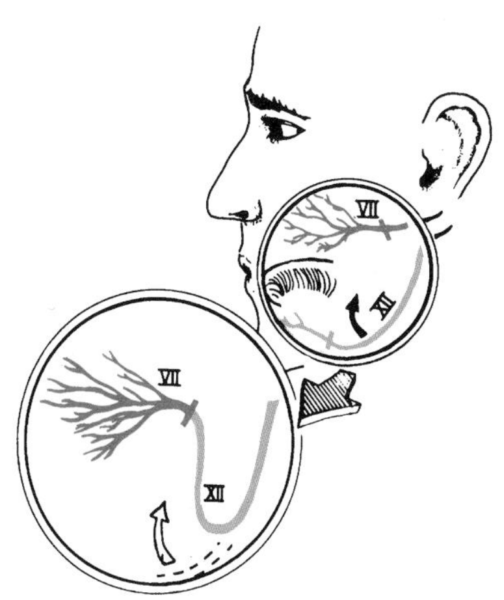

If function has not recovered after a year and electrical tests indicate a dead nerve the choice of treatment lies between plastic surgery to raise the paralysed side of the face with a facial sling, or an operation such as anastomosis between the hypoglossal and facial nerves. *Faciohypoglossal anastomosis* generally produces better results than plastic surgery but it cannot be performed after the muscle fibres have atrophied—a process that usually takes two or three years.

THROAT INFECTIONS

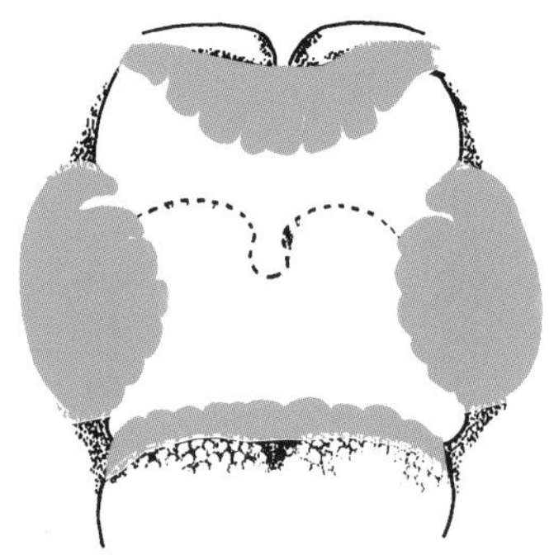

The back of the nose and buccal cavity are encircled by a ring of lymphoid tissue. This (Waldeyer's ring) comprises adenoid tissues in the postnasal space, the pharyngeal tonsils, and the lingual tonsil. Shortly after birth the lymphoid tissue enlarges physiologically and remains enlarged until puberty. In early childhood this tissue plays a part in normal immunological development.

Infection of the throat may either affect the mucosa of the whole of the nasopharynx and oropharynx (pharyngitis) or be localised to the lymphoid tissue, causing tonsillitis.

Acute infections: causes and diagnosis

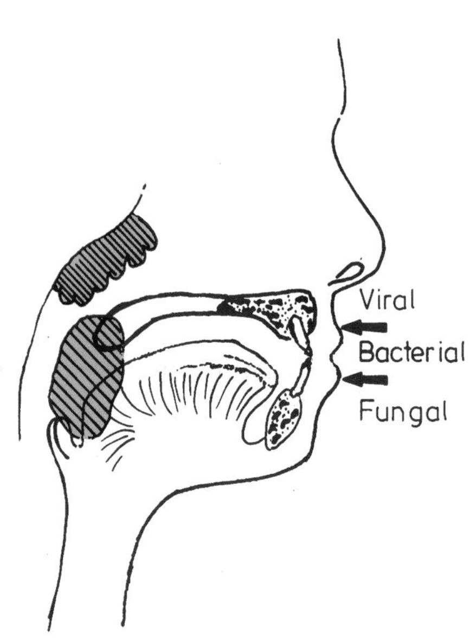

Acute pharyngitis and acute tonsillitis may be due to viral, bacterial, or fungal infection. Half of all infections are viral, caused by the influenza viruses, parainfluenza viruses, adenoviruses, respiratory syncytial virus, and rhinoviruses.

Bacterial infections are usually due to *Streptococcus haemolyticus* and less often to *Str pneumoniae* and *Haemophilus influenzae*. Rare but important causes include diphtheria and gonococcal infection. Secondly syphilis also causes a generalised pharyngitis, with highly infective snail track ulcers. Tuberculosis is a rare cause of pharyngeal infection, usually associated with open pulmonary disease.

Monilia is the most common fungal infection, occurring in debilitated patients and those who have been taking oral antibiotics. It causes white patches. Moniliasis is best treated by sipping nystatin suspension 1 ml four times a day.

Acute tonsillitis, with its typical clinical pattern of fever, malaise, dysphagia, and cervical lymphadenitis, occurs when acute infection is localised to the tonsils. Whenever examination shows membranous exudate diphtheria should be suspected, and urgent treatment with antidiphtheria antitoxin and penicillin should be started before the diagnosis is confirmed bacteriologically. The anginose variety of infectious mononucleosis may also cause a shaggy exudate in the tonsillar region.

The differential diagnosis of any sore throat with ulceration must also include blood dyscrasias and agranulocytosis. Unusual patterns of throat infection and lymphadenopathy should raise suspicion of HIV infection.

Treatment of acute tonsillitis

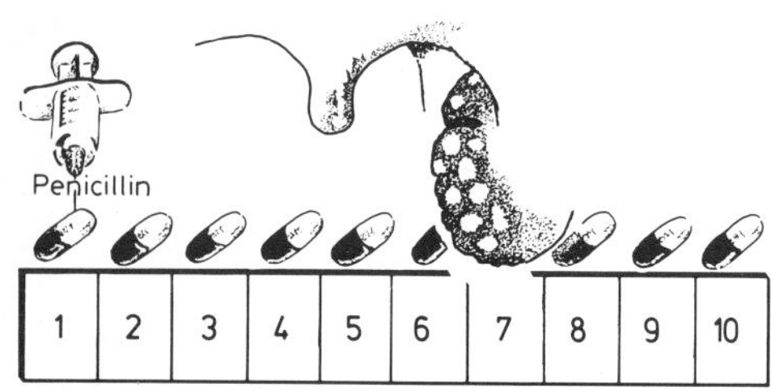

If possible a throat swab should be taken in cases of acute tonsillitis, but antibiotics must be started at once if the infection is severe. Penicillin is the drug of choice and the first dose should, ideally, be given intramuscularly. A course of penicillin should be continued for 10 days, since recrudescence often occurs because organisms persist deep in the crypts. Alternative antibiotics include erythromycin, co-trimoxazole, or Augmentin, (amoxycillin, and clavulanic acid, a β lactamase inhibitor). Ampicillin must not be used for teenagers, because of the high prevalence of glandular fever and the risk of skin rash. Symptomatic treatment involves bed rest, a liquid diet, and soluble aspirin to relieve pain.

Complications of acute infection

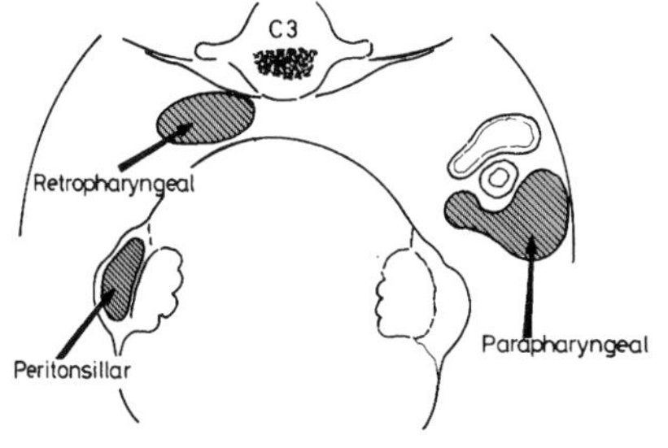

The spread of infection to sites adjacent to the tonsils may cause various abscesses: acute retropharyngeal abscess, peritonsillar abscess, cervical adenitis with abscess formation, parapharyngeal abscess, and Ludwig's angina. Acute otitis media may also be a complication of acute infection of the tonsils and adenoids.

Systemic diseases occur as immunological responses to group A β haemolytic streptococci. They include rheumatic fever, acute glomerulonephritis, and Sydenham's chorea.

Retropharyngeal abscesses

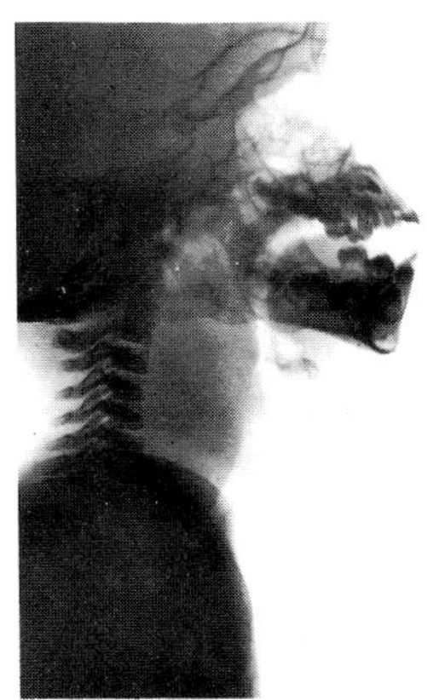

Acute retropharyngeal abscesses are caused by suppurative infection of retropharyngeal lymph nodes, which are present only in babies and young children. The clinical picture is non-specific: the child is feverish, unwell, and fails to eat or drink. Displacement of the posterior pharyngeal wall is not apparent because the whole posterior wall is pushed nearer to the observer than normal. Apart from the help given by finding a high white cell count the diagnosis depends on examining a lateral radiograph of the soft tissue of the neck, which should always be taken when this condition is suspected; this shows increased soft tissue between the vertebral column and the airway. If untreated the abscess is likely to burst through the posterior pharyngeal wall and drown the baby in pus. The abscess has to be incised with the baby in the head down position and the surgeon must be prepared to aspirate large amounts of pus.

Peritonsillar abscess (quinsy)

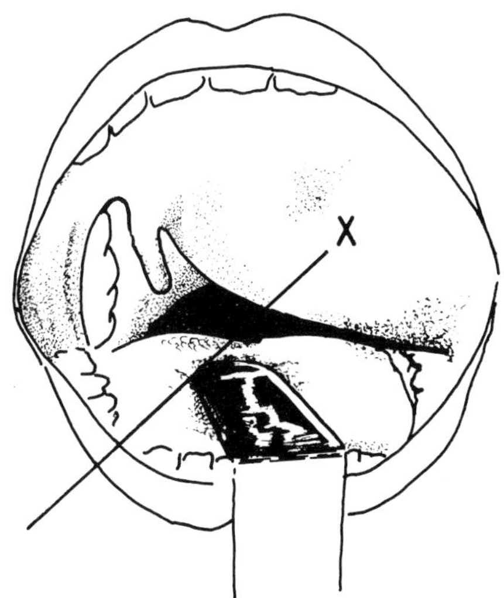

Quinsy occurs when pus accumulates between the tonsil and its bed. The disease is almost always unilateral; the accumulating pus displaces the tonsil medially and backwards so that the swollen soft palate obscures the tonsil. The uvula is displaced across the midline and only the unaffected tonsil is usually visible. Clinically there is a typical picture of tonsillitis, but then difficulty in swallowing increases, trismus develops, and even saliva may not be swallowed. The diagnosis is easily made by observing the oropharynx through the mouth, though access may be difficult because of trismus. When a quinsy is fully developed the mucosa over the pointing abscess is soft to touch.

Conventional treatment to release the pus is to incise the abscess under local anaesthesia with the patient in the sitting position. An alternative is to perform "abscess tonsillectomy" under general anaesthetic. This demands skilled anaesthetic induction since rupture of the quinsy during intubation may result in fatal aspiration of pus. An apparent quinsy is often seen at the stage of cellulitis before the pus has localised, when incision will not help. Instead patients should be admitted for symptomatic relief and treated with large doses of intravenous penicillin. If the swelling abates and the condition resolves antibiotics must be continued for at least 10 days.

Other local complications

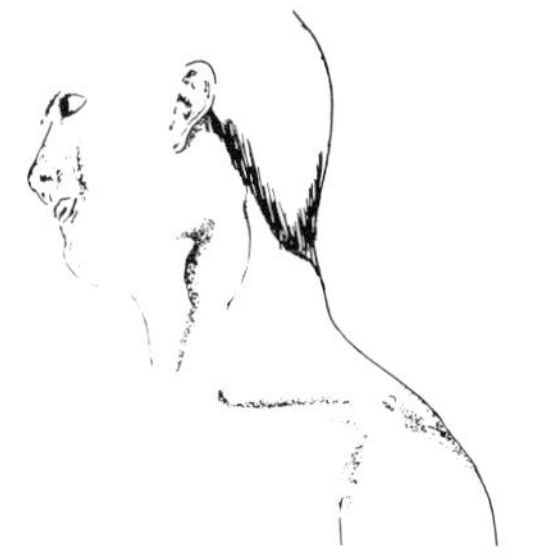

Cervical adenitis suppuration presents after an upper respiratory tract infection in children with a fluctuating tender swelling in the position of the jugulodigastic lymph node. As well as antibiotics, treatment requires incision and drainage of the abscess through the skin of the neck.

Parapharyngeal abscess is a rare complication of tonsillitis. Pus accumulates in the parapharyngeal space lateral to the tonsil bed. Since the large vessels of the neck run through this space the condition may be fatal if the carotid artery ruptures.

Other local complications: very rare today?

Ludwig's angina is also rare. Cellulitis occurs and pus accumulates in the floor of the mouth above and below the mylohyoid muscle. This causes brawny induration of the neck and upward displacement of the tongue, embarrassing respiration. The neck has to be incised to drain pus.

Chronic pharyngitis

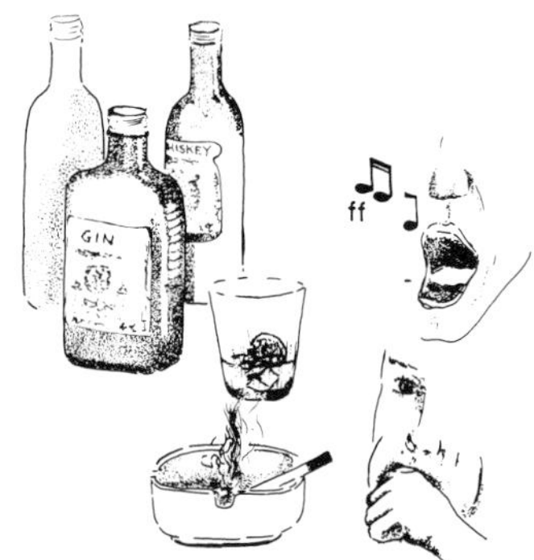

Chronic inflammation of the pharyngeal mucosa is always caused by continuing irritation from another source—chronic sinus infection, chronic mouth breathing because of nasal obstruction, overuse of the voice in shouting and singing, smoking, spirit drinking, coughing, and repeated vomiting. Frequent attacks of acute infection may cause scarring, with enclosure of infected debris in the crypts, and intratonsillar abscesses. This in turn may produce chronic infection in the tonsils.

The offending irritation needs to be prevented, and if the chronically diseased state is harmful the patient may benefit from tonsillectomy.

Tonsillectomy and adenoidectomy

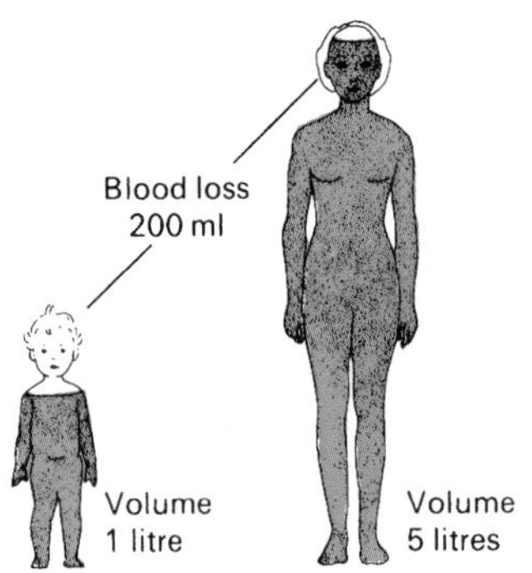

The risks of removing the tonsils and adenoids must be weighed against the disadvantages that the patient will continue to suffer if no operation is performed. The hazards of operation, particularly the risk associated with blood loss, are much greater in small children than in large children or adults because the total blood volume is much less. Much stronger reasons are therefore needed for operating on a child under 4 years or weighing less than 12 kg (blood volume 1 litre).

Indications for adenoidectomy alone

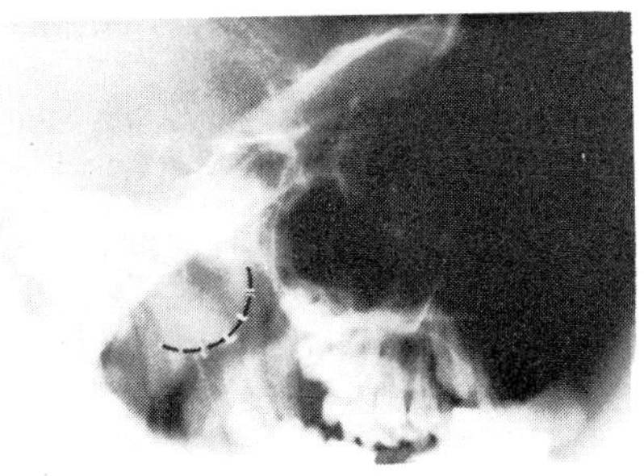

Adenoidectomy alone is indicated for mechanical reasons when enlargement (*a*) causes nasal obstruction with mouth breathing during the daytime and recurrent sore throats because of the drying effect; (*b*) causes gross interference with palatal movement and speech development; (*c*) encroaches on the nasopharyngeal orifice of the Eustachian tube in secretory otitis media or recurrent otitis media. In all these cases preoperative assessment of adenoid size by lateral radiography of the soft tissue of the postnasal space is advisable.

Indications for tonsillectomy and adenoidectomy

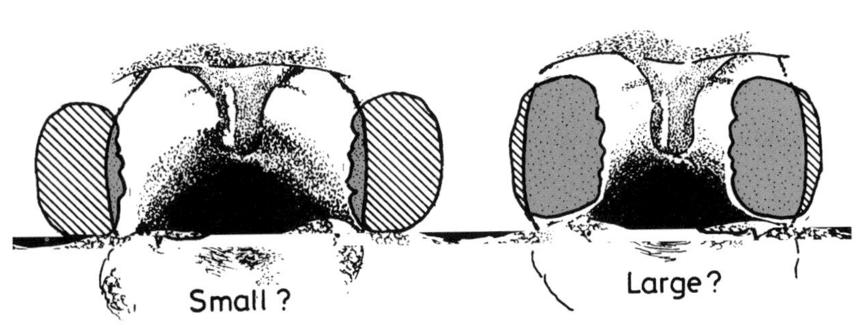

Tonsillar enlargement is great enough to justify tonsillectomy only in *obstructive sleep apnoea*. Tonsils vary in size and in the extent to which they are visible within the pharynx because they vary in their relation to the pillars of the fauces. They normally enlarge after birth and remain enlarged throughout childhood. Tonsils may be considered abnormally large when they have swollen during an attack of acute tonsillitis and have not diminished after recovery. The *obstructive sleep apnoea syndrome* is becoming more often

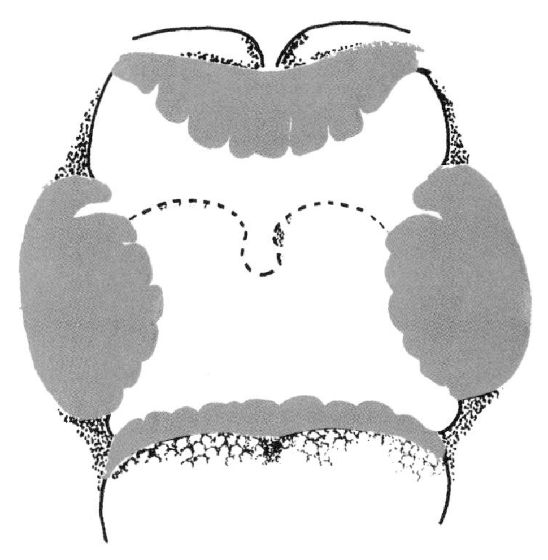

recognised. There is loud snoring at night and cessation of breathing for at least 10 seconds 30 times or more during the night. The diagnosis can be confirmed only by nocturnal studies of blood gas levels, but it may be suspected from observation of the sleeping pattern. It causes daytime lethargy and sleepiness, failure to thrive, pectum excavatum, and, in extreme cases, cor pulmonale.

Since adenoid tissue always shares in the infection, tonsillectomy should be accompanied by adenoidectomy (except in adults whose adenoids have atrophied). The commonest indication for tonsillectomy is recurrent attacks of acute bacterial tonsillitis. The critical number of attacks of tonsillitis depends on age. Viral infection is particularly common in children in their first two years at school, but after this tonsillectomy should be considered if there are three or four attacks a year for over two years. In adults repeated attacks of tonsillitis over more than six months or even one attack of a quinsy is a strong indication, since further attacks are almost inevitable.

Tonsillectomy may be considered (*a*) in children with recurrent sore throats with lymphadenitis; (*b*) for recurrent acute suppurative otitis media; (*c*) for the obstructive sleep apnoea syndrome; (*d*) in patients with a history of the systemic complications of haemolytic streptococcal infection; and (*e*) for the rare condition of chronic tonsillar infection in patients suffering from disorders such as psoriasis and immune complex disease affecting the eyes—removing the tonsils may improve the general disorder.

Hazards of operation

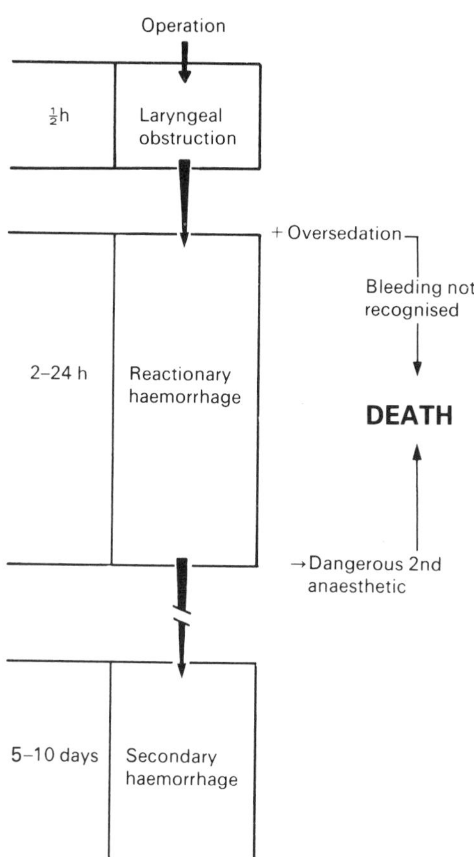

In general, dissection is preferable to guillotine extraction for removing the tonsils. Adenoid tissue is removed by curettes. Skilled general anaesthesia is essential, and most surgeons prefer to operate on patients who have been intubated as an added protection to the airway.

The main hazards of operation are inhalation of blood during operation; respiratory obstruction due to laryngeal spasm immediately after the operation; postoperative haemorrhage; and accidental damage to neighbouring structures.

The most dangerous postoperative bleeding occurs in the first 24 hours after operation. Deaths have followed because bleeding has not been recognised owing to excessive sedation or because operative attempts to stop the flow have necessitated anaesthesia in a patient with a depleted blood volume and a full stomach. Secondary haemorrhage caused by infection of the tonsillar bed seven to 10 days after operation is much less dangerous.

Damage to the palate and uvula should not occur in skilled hands. Occasionally teeth may be chipped or displaced and the Eustachian cushion may be damaged by the curette. Theoretically the anterior surface of the cervical vertebrae and even the internal carotid artery are at risk.

It is undesirable to expose any young child to operation, but much of the emotional disturbance can be removed if the mother is admitted with the child.

In deciding whether or not to perform tonsillectomy and adenoidectomy the surgeon will find the history and the general practitioner's records more useful than examination. Not too much attention need be paid to the appearance and size of the tonsils: it is more important to try to distinguish between viral and bacterial causes of infection and to assess the severity of the attacks.

HOARSENESS AND STRIDOR

Hoarseness and stridor in children

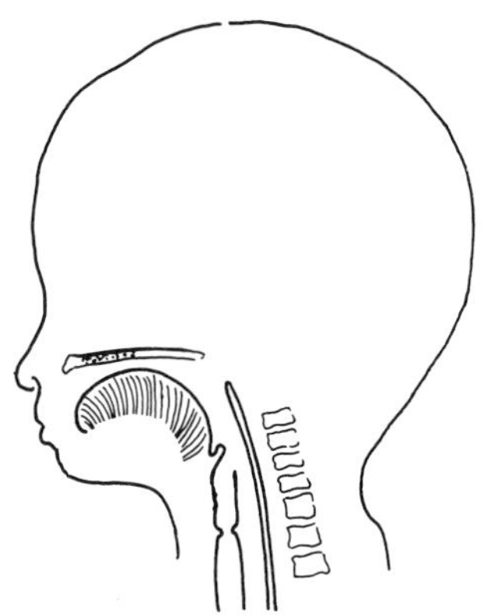

Obstruction of the airway in the small larynx and trachea is much more rapid and life threatening than in the adult. Stridor indicates airway obstruction and it may be associated with voice changes, swallowing difficulties causing failure to gain weight, and respiratory infections. More serious signs of obstruction include cyanosis and pallor, dilatation of the nares, recession of the soft chest wall, downward plunging of the trachea with respiration, and use of the accessory muscles of respiration.

Causes of obstruction include (*a*) congenital abnormalities of the larynx—laryngomalacia, laryngeal stenosis, rare tumours; (*b*) inflammatory conditions such as acute laryngitis, acute epiglottitis, laryngotracheobronchitis; (*c*) neurological abnormalities—vagal or recurrent laryngeal nerve paralysis; (*d*) trauma to the larynx—birth injuries, intubation injury; (*e*) inhalation of foreign bodies.

Neonatal stridor

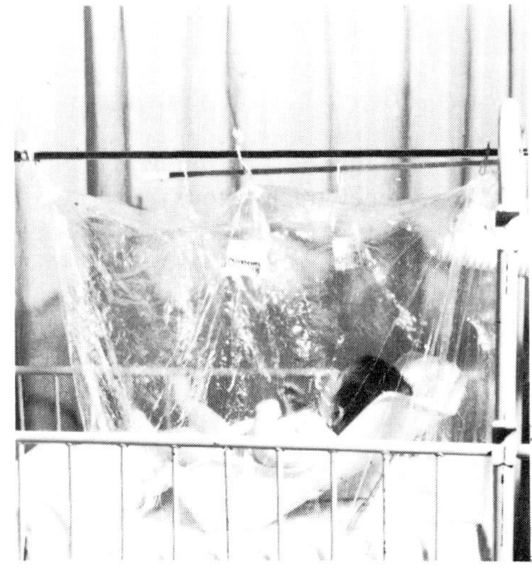

Assessing stridor in the neonate demands skilled examination of the larynx. An experienced paediatric laryngologist will usually perform the examination under general anaesthesia. The urgency of referral for examination depends on the degree of associated respiratory obstruction and failure to thrive.

Respiration may be helped by nursing the infant in a croupette, which provides a cool, moist atmosphere. The need to preserve the airway may necessitate either endotracheal intubation or tracheostomy while the cause is being treated in hospital.

Laryngomalacia (congenital laryngeal stridor) causes respiratory stridor that is particularly noticeable when the child is asleep. The noise persists for the first four to five years of life and the infant is slow to gain weight. There is no specific treatment. Problems may arise when there is incidental laryngeal infection.

Laryngeal paralysis from birth accounts for a quarter of the cases of stridor in infancy; it is probably due to stretching of the vagus nerve during a difficult delivery. The condition is usually associated with feeding difficulties, and again there is no specific treatment.

Congenital narrowing of the larynx, by webs between the cords or by restriction of the subglottic space with thickening of the cricoid arch, presents difficult laryngological problems requiring skilled surgery.

Infective causes

Diphtheria is rare but should not be excluded

Stridor in a child with a previously adequate airway is usually caused by infective swelling, but inhaled foreign bodies, trauma from ingesting corrosive agents, and allergic oedema must be considered.

Acute laryngitis causes classical "croup" with a croupy cough and stridor at night. This common condition is usually managed at home with the standard treatment for upper respiratory tract infections supported by nursing in a humidified environment. If dyspnoea supervenes the more dangerous infective conditions must be considered—laryngotracheobronchitis, acute epiglottitis, and (rarely) diphtheria.

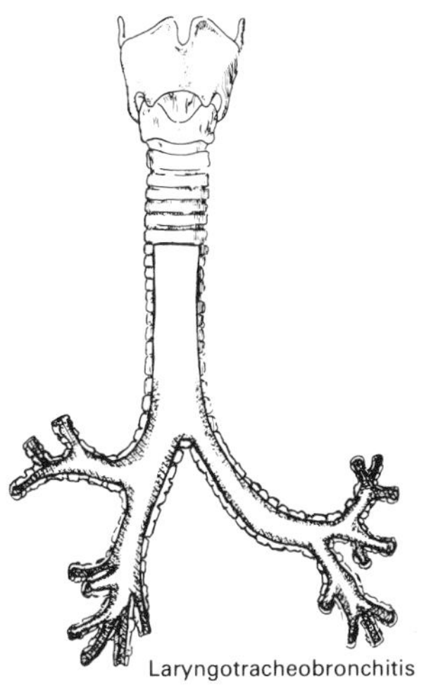
Laryngotracheobronchitis

Laryngotracheobronchitis affects children aged 6 months to 3 years. In parts of the world where measles is common the measles virus is an important cause of laryngotracheobronchitis. Otherwise it is usually caused by the parainfluenza or respiratory syncytial viruses. The disorder is characterised by respiratory obstruction caused by narrowing of the subglottic airway and exudation into the trachea and bronchi of thick tenacious material. Initially it is indistinguishable from acute laryngitis with inspiratory stridor, but dyspnoea then increases with a rising temperature and dehydration. Referral to hospital is essential, where the throat and larynx must be examined with great care because of the risk of laryngeal spasm with total respiratory obstruction and cardiac arrest.

Treatment may often be expectant at first, with nursing in a croupette. Adequate intravenous fluids are essential, and antibiotics are usually given. If such treatment fails, as shown by a rising respiratory rate and increasing obstruction, the tenacious secretions need to be removed from the bronchi. It may be necessary to leave an endotracheal tube in place or to perform a tracheostomy.

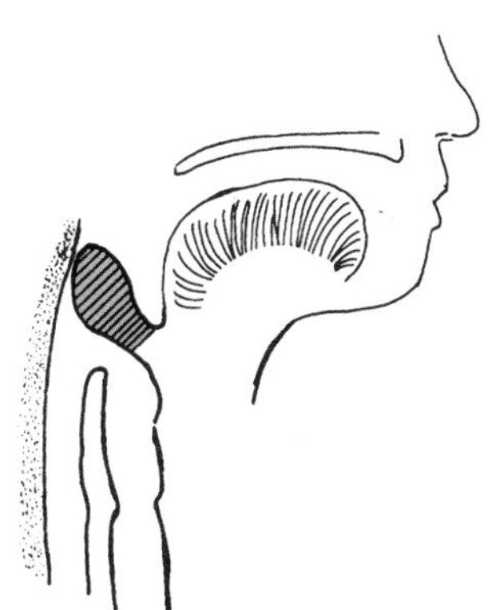

Acute epiglottitis is a serious, often fatal, infection caused by *Haemophilus influenzae* type B, which produces localised oedema of the epiglottis and supraglottic larynx. Initially there is severe dysphagia and a high temperature. Rapidly developing respiratory obstruction is more noticeable than stridor. When epiglottitis is suspected blood culture may yield the infecting organism more readily than a throat swab. The throat must be examined in the operating theatre, by an experienced otolaryngologist, and an anaesthetist. Under no circumstances should attempted examination, even with a tongue depressor, take place in the accident and emergency department, since respiratory obstruction may ensue. Urgent relief for the airway is often needed and specific treatment is usually intravenous ampicillin together with steroids.

If there is a possibility of diphtheria, suggested by the typical pseudomembrane in the throat, antitoxin as well as penicillin should be given as soon as possible.

Relieving severe respiratory obstruction in children

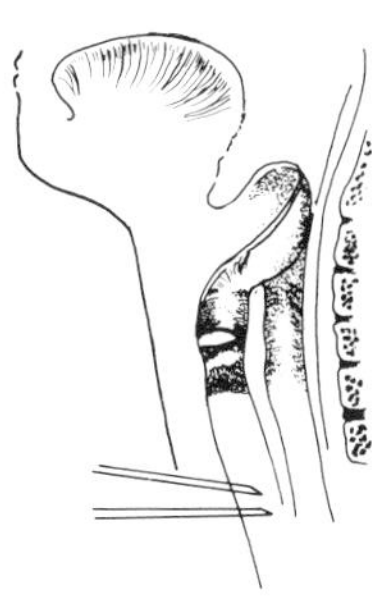

The method of relieving obstruction will depend on the facilities available and the skill of the staff. Emergency tracheostomy is a difficult procedure with a high mortality. Intubation with a soft endotracheal tube is often tried but may prove impossible. If the instruments are to hand the laryngoscope used to try intubation may provide access for a bronchoscope. Tracheostomy may then be performed safely. If these facilities are not available an airway can be provided by inserting one or more small needles straight into the trachea or by using so called "minitrachs."

Hoarseness and stridor in the adult

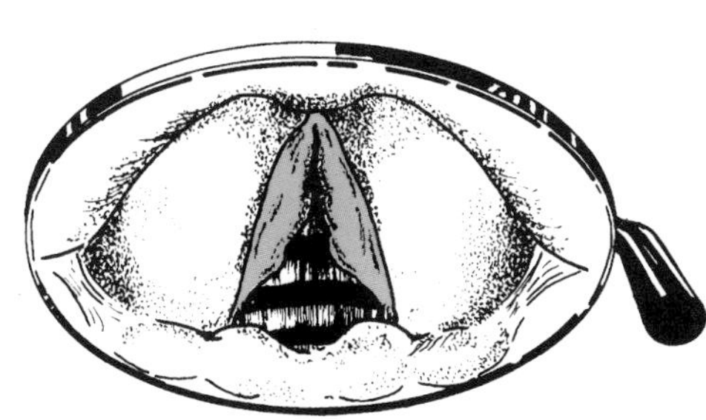

In the adult laryngeal problems more often cause voice changes than respiratory obstruction. Hoarseness occurs whenever a normal smooth vocal cord is not brought firmly into apposition with its fellow. The causes are irregularities of the surface of the cord or neuromuscular disorders affecting their movement.

Acute hoarseness may be caused by acute infective laryngitis; acute trauma from shouting, coughing, vomiting, or inhaling noxious fumes; or allergic swelling. Chronic hoarseness—arbitrarily defined as a change in the voice lasting more than three weeks—may be due to persistence of any of the acute causes; chronic laryngitis; vocal cord paralysis; neoplasia; and, rarely, arthritis of the laryngeal joints.

Chronic laryngitis is usually caused by continuing irritation of the laryngeal mucosa. This is often due to vocal abuse, particularly when straining the voice during an attack of acute laryngitis, with

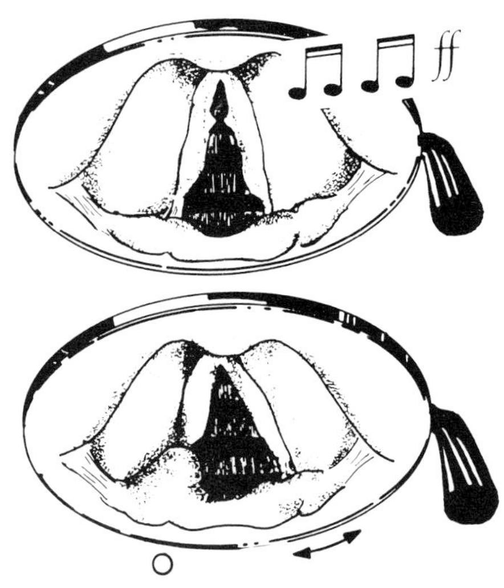

submucosal haemorrhage and vocal cord oedema. Smoking, inhalation of spirits, desiccation during mouth breathing, and frequent coughing or vomiting also cause persisting irritation. Specific infections of the larynx by tuberculosis and tertiary syphilis are also possible causes. Changes in the cords include persistent oedema of both or the development of polypoid swellings. Vocal cord nodules ("singer's nodes") occur particularly under certain forms of voice strain and appear as tiny fibrous nodules at the junction of the anterior third and posterior two thirds of both vocal cords. Chronic laryngitis may also be associated with keratotic changes in the surface of the cords, producing white patches (leucoplakia), which are sometimes premalignant. "Contact" ulcers sometimes occur at the posterior ends of the cords from trauma of one arytenoid hitting the other.

Vocal cord paralysis is usually caused by damage to the recurrent laryngeal nerve. An important cause is neoplasia affecting the left nerve at the hilum of the lung. It may also result from trauma during thyroidectomy and from any cause of neuritis. Often no cause can be found.

Neoplasms of the larynx

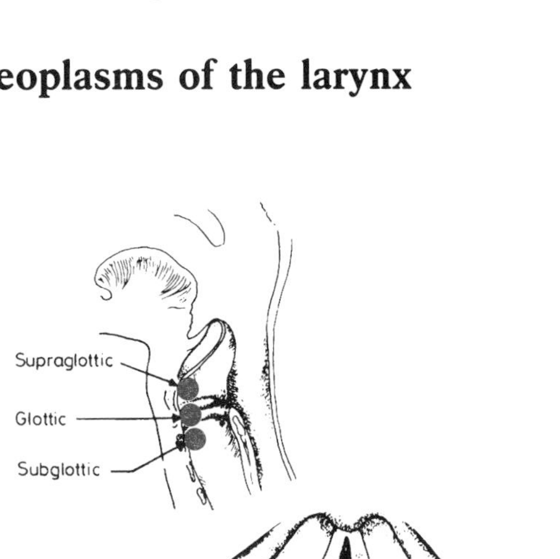

Among neoplasms of the larynx the malignant tumours are usually squamous cell carcinomas, which are commoner in men than in women. They may arise from the vocal cords (glottic) or from above or below them (supraglottic or subglottic). Glottic carcinomas have the best prognosis because they cause hoarseness earlier (and thus present earlier) and spread to the lymphatic nodes in the neck much later than the other two types. Carcinomas of the pyriform fossa cause hoarseness by invading the muscles of the larynx, but this occurs late in the development of the tumour, although early in its presentation.

All patients with hoarseness persisting for over three weeks should be referred for indirect laryngoscopy to diagnose the cause of the voice change. Skilled laryngologists rarely fail to see the larynx well with a mirror, but the information may need to be supplemented by fibreoptic endoscopy as an outpatient, or by direct laryngoscopy under anaesthetic. This also offers an opportunity to biopsy abnormal tissue. Further investigations may include computed tomography of the larynx and a chest radiograph.

Treatment

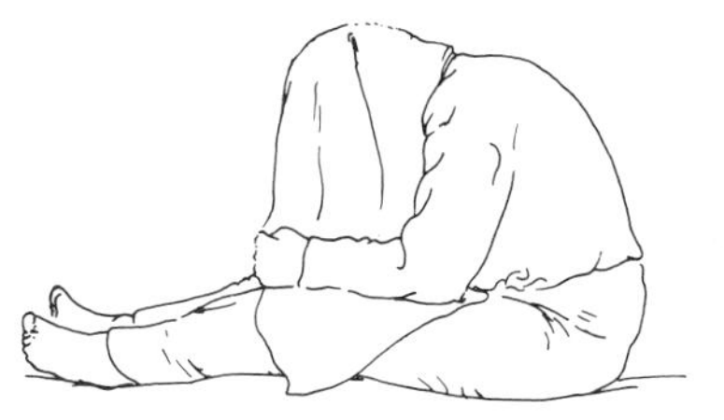

In general chronic laryngitis must be treated with voice rest and elimination of the irritating factors. Humidification of the home may be useful, as may steam inhalations with Friar's balsam. Innocent swellings of the larynx may need removing by microlaryngoscopy using the binocular microscope. Malignant tumours are treated by combinations of external irradiation, cytotoxic drugs, and surgery.

A weak voice from cord paralysis may be helped by injection of teflon paste to displace the vocal fold medially.

Relieving airway obstruction in the adult

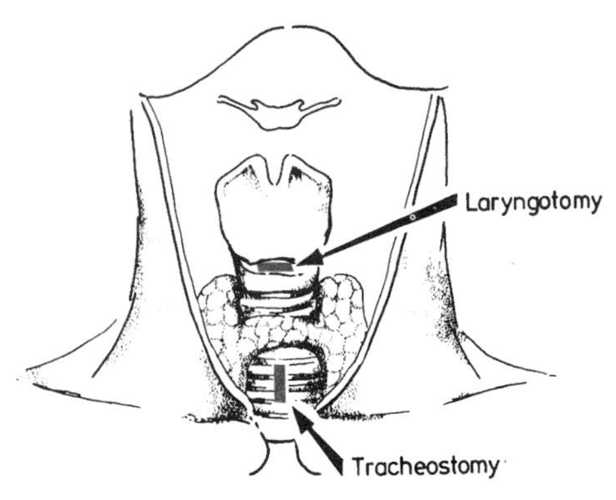

Airway obstruction in the adult may result from gradual narrowing by large exfoliative tumours, bilateral recurrent laryngeal paralysis, and inhalation of foreign bodies—particularly lumps of food aspirated into the larynx. Urgent relief of laryngeal obstruction is best achieved by laryngotomy. An incision is made over the cricothyroid membrane and any available tube inserted. This procedure is much simpler and safer in unskilled hands than tracheostomy, since the cricothyroid membrane is just below the surface of the skin, whereas the trachea plunges deep to the vascular thyroid gland as it descends.

In hospital the respiratory obstruction of a slowly developing tumour will usually be managed by tracheostomy. Respiratory embarrassment from bilateral recurrent laryngeal nerve paralysis can be helped by removing the arytenoid and displacing the cord laterally (arytenoidectomy).

DIFFICULTY IN SWALLOWING

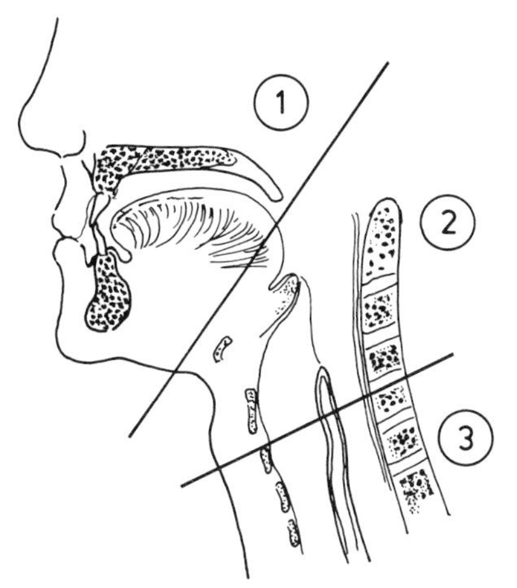

The commonest causes of *acute* dysphagia are inflammatory disorders and foreign bodies, which are discussed in other chapters. When dysphagia is *chronic* the doctor must first identify the stage of swallowing that is affected. Difficulty with the first two stages of swallowing—passing the bolus to the back of the throat and initiating the swallowing reflex—is caused by neuromuscular disorders and is relatively rare. Dysphagia after the initiation of the involuntary swallowing reflex is much more common and is usually caused by lesions within the laryngopharynx and oesophagus, though, rarely, the oesophageal lumen may be compressed from outside or deranged by diseases of its wall as in scleroderma. The neuromuscular disorders that disrupt the first two stages of swallowing include motor neurone disease, multiple sclerosis, paralysis of the lower bulbar nerves after posterior cranial fossa operations or infarction of the medulla, and infection of the bulbar neurones in acute anterior poliomyelitis.

Is the cause organic?

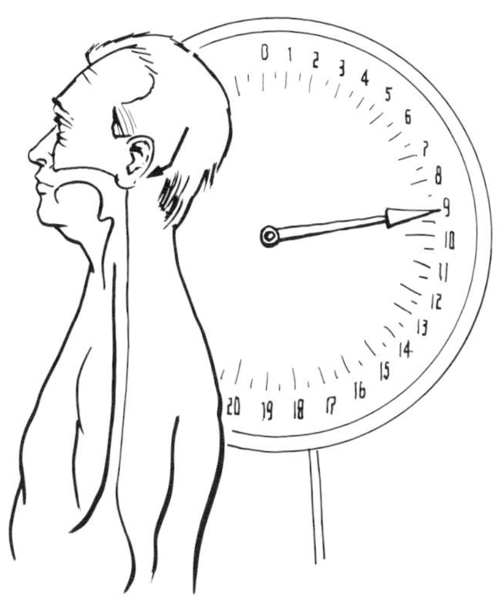

If a patient with dysphagia has lost weight, has pain referred to the ear on swallowing, has undergone a voice change, or suffers regurgitation of food into the mouth an organic cause for the dysphagia must be sought. Often, however, he or she will complain of a sensation of a lump in the throat for which no organic cause can be found. This disorder—sometimes called "globus hystericus"—most often affects women and may be due to spasm of the cricopharyngeus muscle. It should be suspected whenever the sensation of a lump lying centrally in the throat at the level of the larynx persists for several months without weight loss, obstruction to swallowing, or abnormal clinical findings. It may be associated with gastro-oesophageal reflux.

If the history suggests an organic cause for dysphagia during the third or reflex stage of swallowing the important causes to consider are postcricoid carcinoma, other malignant tumours of the laryngopharynx, hypopharyngeal diverticula, benign strictures of the oesophagus, achalasia of the cardia, and carcinoma of the oesophagus.

In many of these cases, including those of benign stricture and carcinoma, the patient might often be referred to a general or thoracic surgeon rather than an otolaryngologist.

Postcricoid carcinoma

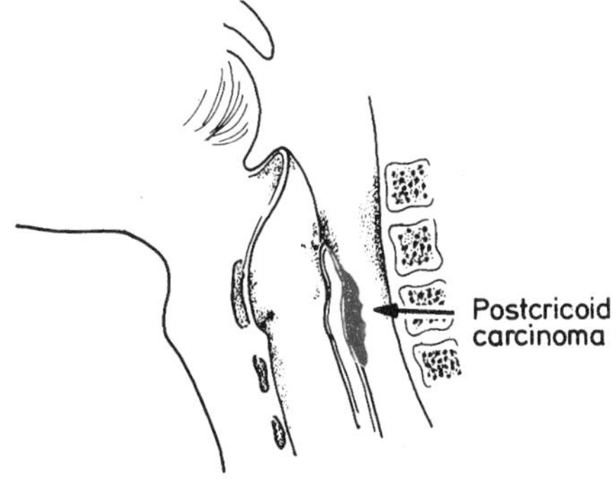

Postcricoid carcinoma invariably occurs in middle aged women who suffer from chronic iron deficiency anaemia. The dysphagia, together with the other features of iron deficiency anaemia—koilonychya, glossitis, and angular stomatitis—constitute the Paterson Brown-Kelly syndrome. The development of malignant neoplasia is preceded for some years by the formation of a fibrous postcricoid web, immediately under atrophic postcricoid mucosa. In the early stages, before neoplasia develops, the patient must be treated by restoring serum iron concentrations to normal and maintaining them. Postcricoid webs may be dilated through an endoscope.

Other malignant tumours of the laryngopharynx

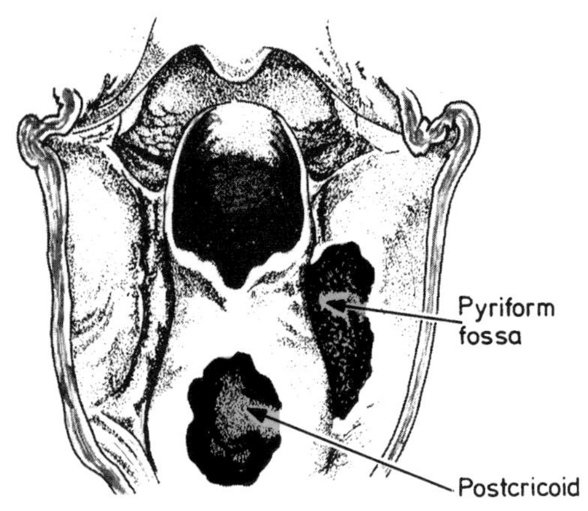

Other tumours, particularly those of the pyriform fossa, are far commoner in men than in women and do not cause dysphagia until they become large because the food channel is much wider at the level of the pyriform fossa. An elderly man with a tumour of the laryngopharynx would probably have progressive hoarseness, pain referred to the ear, and cervical lymphadenopathy.

As with postcricoid carcinomas, curative treatment includes radiotherapy, sometimes combined with cytotoxic drugs. If the larynx and surrounding pharynx has to be removed there are several reconstructive techniques available to establish continuity between the oropharynx and oesophagus. In many cases the chance of cure is so low that treatment should be considered only palliative.

Pharyngeal pouches

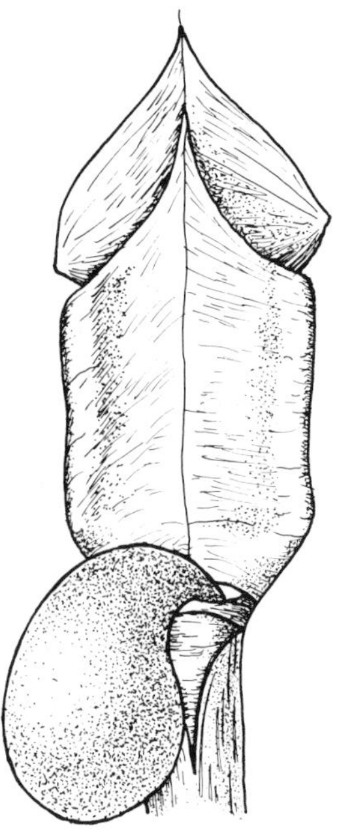

Pharyngeal pouches—or hypopharyngeal diverticula—usually develop in middle aged to elderly men. The pharyngeal mucosa between the upper and lower parts of the inferior constrictor muscle (thyropharyngeus and cricopharyngeus) becomes herniated through the dehiscence of Killian, in the midline posteriorly. As the pharyngeal pouch enlarges, food is regurgitated into the mouth, and this may be provoked by pressing on the skin of the neck over the pouch. Intermittent overspill of the content of the pouch into the larynx causes coughing and, sometimes, recurrent aspiration pneumonia and pneumonitis. If the pouch grows very large it becomes the preferential channel for the passage of food, and when it is full its pressure on the oesophagus completely obstructs swallowing. Relief is achieved only by emptying the pouch. Small pouches may need no treatment or only simple dilatation of the postcricoid region with an endoscope, but larger pouches may have to be removed by external operation. A valuable alternative, particularly in a frail patient, is surgical endoscopic division of the wall between the pouch and the oesophagus by diathermy (Dohlman's operation).

Benign strictures of the oesophagus and carcinoma of the oesophagus

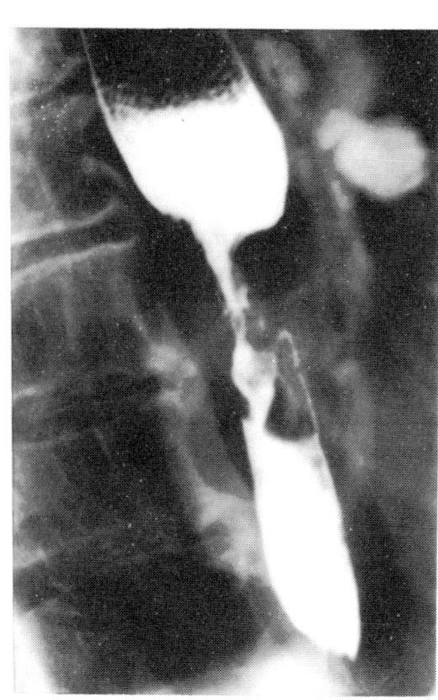

Benign strictures may develop from chronic oesophagitis and are often associated with longstanding gastric reflux. They can be treated by endoscopic dilatation combined with medical measures to prevent gastric reflux and gastric acid secretion.

Carcinoma of the oesophagus presents, usually in elderly men, with a story of progressive dysphagia and loss of weight. The typical radiographic barium swallow appearance of an irregular stricture should suggest the diagnosis, which has to be confirmed histologically on material removed endoscopically. Histological examination is also needed for the much rarer benign tumours of the oesophagus, such as leiomyoma.

Achalasia of the cardia

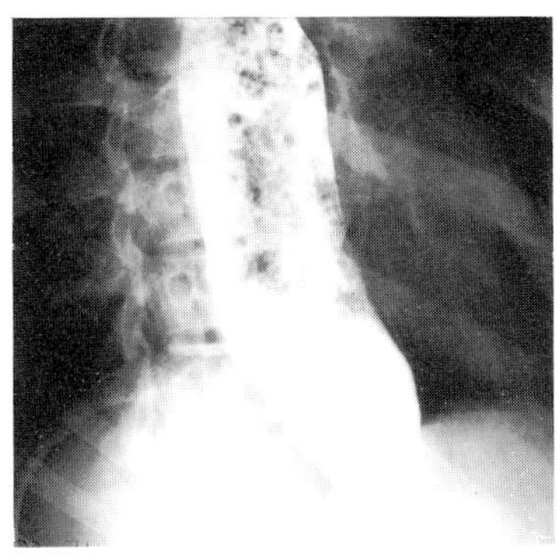

Achalasia is a neuromuscular disorder preventing free passage from the oesophagus to the stomach, with gross dilatation of the oesophagus above. The clinical picture is similar to that of benign stricture or carcinoma of the oesophagus, but there are often periods of remission. The diagnosis may be suggested by the radiographic appearance of a barium swallow but must be confirmed by endoscopy. Achalasia of the cardia is treated either by stretching the lower oesophageal sphincter with a hydrostatic bag or by Heller's operation (cardiomyotomy), in which the oesophageal musculature at the cardio-oesophageal junction is incised down to the mucosa.

Assessment and examination

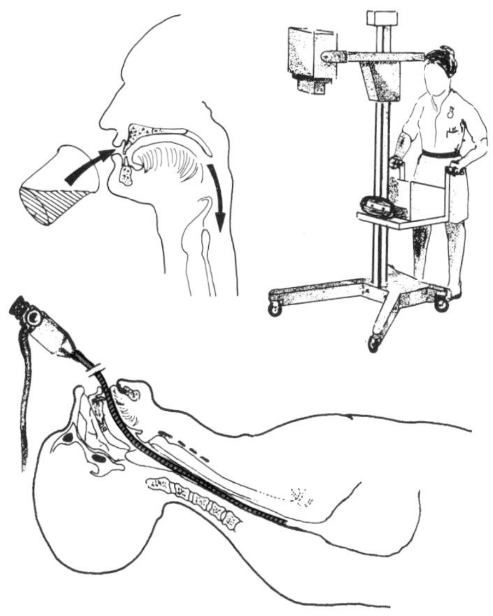

Correct diagnosis demands a careful clinical history. Nevertheless, this may be misleading about the level of the lesion since low oesophageal obstruction often produces a sense of blockage much higher. Examination of the pharynx and palate may show impaired mobility. Pooling of food or saliva in the pyriform fossa, seen with a laryngeal mirror, is always a sign of physical obstruction.

A lateral radiograph of the neck is useful since it may show thickening of the soft tissues between the larynx and vertebral column in postcricoid carcinoma. Barium swallow examination is usually essential, and observation by the radiologist with video recording during the swallow will provide far more valuable information than the still photograph.

Further investigation of any abnormality requires endoscopy. This is now often performed with fibreoptic endoscopes, which offer less risk of damage to the oesophageal mucosa than do the traditional rigid large bore oesophagoscopes.

In assessing a patient with dysphagia it is important to decide how far to investigate. If there is any doubt that an organic lesion might be overlooked then barium swallow and endoscopy must be carried out.

Palliative relief of dysphagia

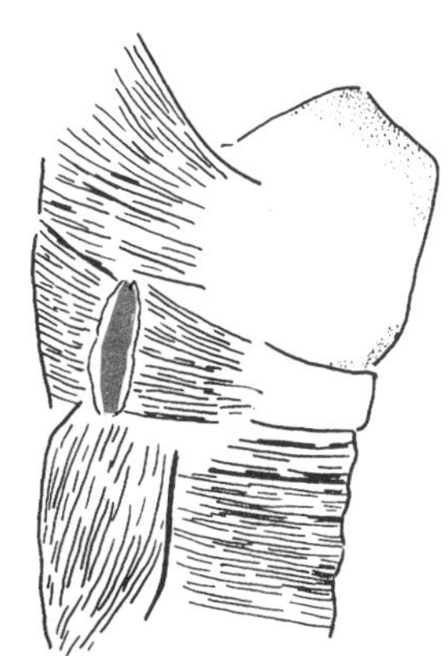

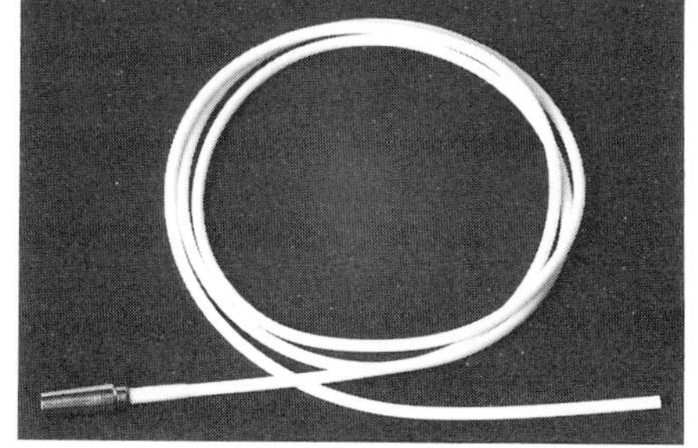

Cricopharyngeal myotomy—external division of the cricopharyngeus muscles down to the hypopharyngeal mucosa—is helpful in neuromuscular disorders that affect the oropharynx and laryngopharynx; it is particularly useful in managing severe dysphagia in motor neurone disease. It is effective particularly when the blockage is at the level of the cricopharyngeus rather than when the main difficulty is in passing the bolus from the mouth to the pharynx.

The dysphagia of inoperable carcinoma of the oesophagus may often be helped by passing a metal or plastic tube through an endoscope.

Nutrition in severe dysphagia may require passage of a nasogastric tube or a gastrostomy. Very fine nasogastric tubes, causing minimal discomfort to the patient, allow a high energy diet to be administered by continuous or intermittent infusion. Gastrostomy is occasionally preferable in a patient who can leave hospital and manage his own food intake, but it does not ease the distressing inability to swallow saliva that is suffered by many patients. Salivary secretion can sometimes be reduced by giving anticholinergic drugs (though these cause side effects) or by denervation of the salivary glands (tympanic neurectomy and chorda tympani section).

Overspill into the larynx may be helped by partially closing the entry to the larynx with the epiglottis—epiglottopexy. Sometimes a cuffed tracheostomy tube is needed.

NASAL OBSTRUCTION

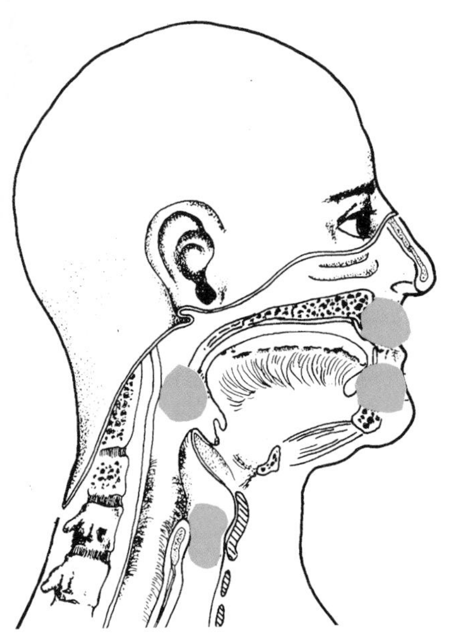

Acute shortlasting nasal obstruction is familiar as a symptom of the common cold and other upper respiratory tract viruses, trauma, and allergic reactions. Some patients, however, suffer chronic nasal obstruction, which is the subject of this chapter.

Chronic nasal obstruction in childhood is most often caused by enlarged adenoids or by vasomotor rhinitis. Rare causes include congenital choanal atresia and tumours of the postnasal space (such as the nasopharyngeal angiofibroma).

Chronic nasal obstruction in the adult is usually caused either by a deflection of the nasal septum or by vasomotor rhinitis and the mucosal swellings which vasomotor rhinitis may produce. A less common cause is chronic sinusitis (which is dealt with in the chapter on paranasal sinus diseases). Rare possibilities include benign and malignant tumours of the nose, paranasal sinuses, and nasopharynx and bacterially induced granulomatous diseases (tuberculosis, syphilis, leprosy). Iatrogenic nasal obstruction produced by topical vasoconstrictors—rhinitis medicamentosa—is so common that it deserves special mention.

The harmful effects of long standing nasal obstruction include chronic pharyngitis, chronic laryngitis, irritation of the gums, distortion of speech, and snoring at night. Temporary nasal obstruction is normal, as is alternation of obstruction between the nasal passages, but people vary greatly in their tolerance of a blocked nose.

Common causes

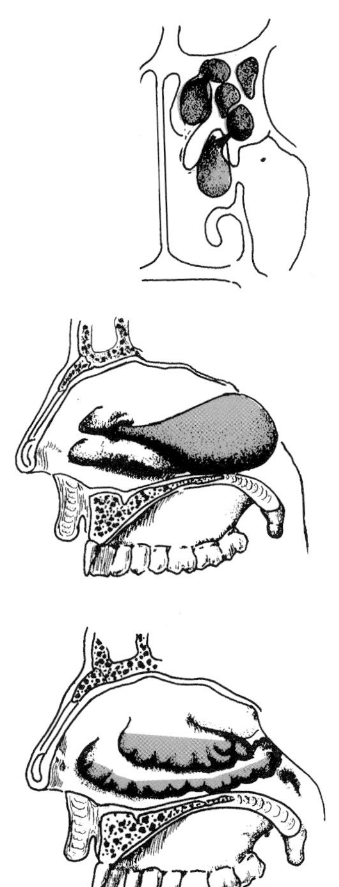

Vasomotor rhinitis, the commonest cause of persisting nasal obstruction in both children and adults, is a disorder of the normal control of the shrinking and swelling of the nasal mucosa whereby it exercises its air conditioning function. The cause may be allergic in a person sensitive to external allergens. It will be seasonal when allergens such as grass pollen persist for short periods at the same time each year, or perennial when allergens like the house dust mite are constantly present. When allergic, vasomotor rhinitis is often associated in childhood with infantile eczema, allergic asthma, and a family history of atopy, and the nasal obstruction is dominated by sneezing and rhinorrhoea.

Often vasomotor rhinitis is not due to any recognisable allergen but is provoked either by external irritating changes of humidity and temperature and non-specific chemical irritants in the atmosphere, or by internal endocrine and emotional factors. Longlasting oedema of the nasal mucosa produces redundant lumps and folds. These may take the form of ethmoid polyps, antrochoanal polyps, and swellings or fringes of the turbinates.

Ethmoid nasal polyps are swellings of the lining of ethmoid cells protruding into the nose. Constriction at the ostium of the cell increases the oedema within the polyp so that it expands within the nasal cavity.

Antrochoanal polyps are much rarer polyps arising from a maxillary antrum; they pass through its ostium backwards to the posterior choana. Since they can develop only from an antrum too small to accommodate its swollen mucosa, they are commoner in children and adolescents than in adults.

Swellings also appear at the posterior end of the inferior turbinates and "moriform fringes" develop from the lower borders of either the middle or inferior turbinates.

Iatrogenic obstruction—Rhinitis medicamentosa results from the treatment of persisting obstruction with nasal decongestant

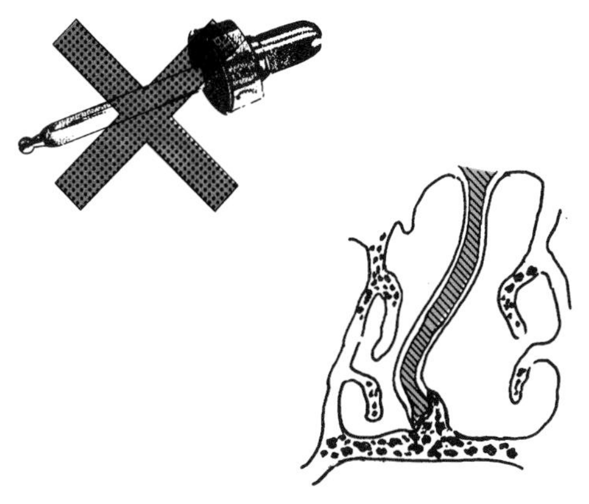

drops or sprays. All these decongestants harm the mucosa if they are used for more than a week at a time. They cause severe vasoconstriction with possible damage by anoxia, followed by a period of rebound engorgement and mucosal oedema which can be relieved only by further administration of the spray. Repeated application produces a swollen red mucosa which eventually becomes rubbery and unresponsive to the decongestant. These sprays are therefore potentially addicting and should be prescribed only when the cause of the nasal obstruction is likely to abate within a week or so. Some systemic drugs, including reserpine and tricyclic antidepressants, may cause nasal stuffiness.

Adenoid enlargement is the other common cause of nasal obstruction in childhood. This has been discussed earlier (see page 32).

A deviated nasal septum is rarely seen in childhood, but 20% or more of adults develop a deflection sufficient to obstruct one nasal passage. This occurs either as developmental asymmetry, particularly in long thin noses, or as a result of injury.

Assessment of the child with a blocked nose

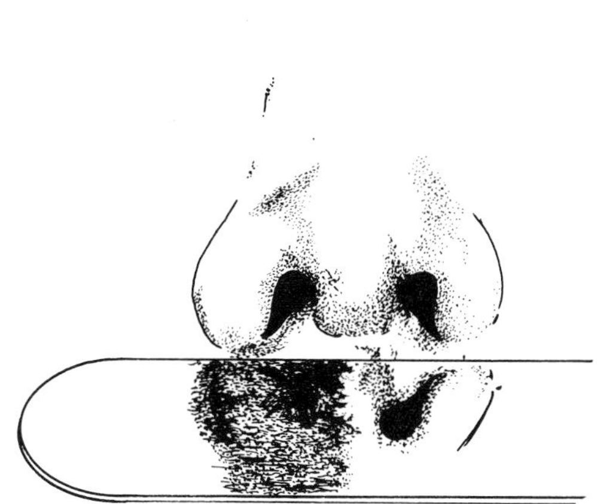

A careful history will tell the doctor the degree of disturbance caused by the obstruction—whether the child breathes through the mouth all the time during the day, whether eating is noisy and speech affected, or whether the concern is mainly snoring at night (see sleep apnoea, page 32). The history will also indicate the relationship of nasal symptoms to possible allergic causes and whether the symptoms are associated with the sneezing that invariably occurs when the cause is allergic.

The doctor must decide whether the child's nose is truly obstructed, since some children keep their mouths open while breathing nasally. The issue can be resolved by holding a shiny speculum under the nose and observing condensation during expiration. This is a useful test for recognising whether one or both nasal passages are obstructed. If only one is completely blocked the rare possibility of unilateral posterior choanal atresia must be considered. Next, examination of the anterior nares may show the oedematous mucosa expected in vasomotor rhinitis. This is often pale mauve. In childhood the inferior turbinates sometimes become persistently oedematous, with large dependent fringes; but other polyoid swellings are unusual.

If the anterior nares are clear, indicating obstruction further back, a lateral radiograph of the postnasal space may be useful, since it can show the degree of adenoid enlargement.

Suspicion of allergy may be followed by skin testing in an attempt to identify the provoking allergens. This is of less practical value than formerly as desensitisation is no longer practised.

The dangers of decongestant drops and sprays have already been described. In the child doctors must decide whether treatment is needed or whether reassurance of the parents will suffice. They should remember that adenoid tissue will atrophy around the time of puberty and that apparent disturbance of sleep by nasal obstruction is often of more concern to the parent than to the child. Adenoidectomy has already been discussed in an earlier chapter.

Assessment of nasal obstruction in the adult

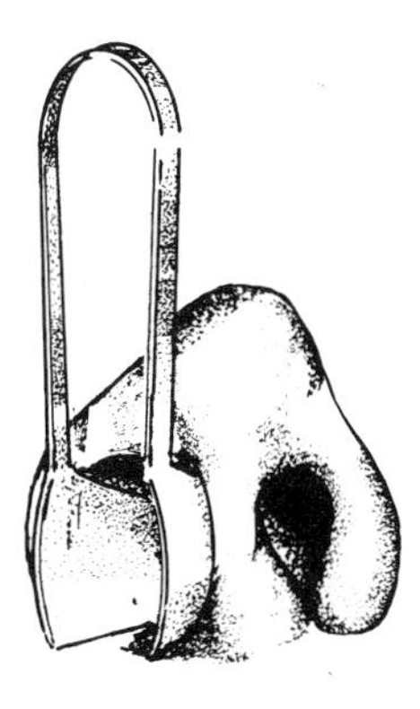

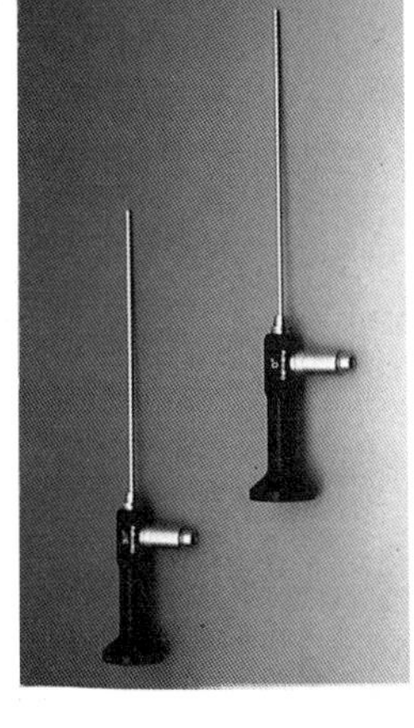

Assessing obstruction in the adult also entails attention to the degree of disturbance; the duration and pattern of the symptom; and whether obstruction affects both nostrils, one continuously, or alternates from one to the other. Constant obstruction of only one side of the nose strongly suggests a deflected nasal septum or, much more rarely, an antrochoanal polyp.

Examination of the adult nose with a speculum and with Hopkin's rod-lens telescopes, and of the postnasal space with a mirror, usually suggests the diagnosis. The response of the mucosa to a vasoconstrictor spray can provide valuable information, and abnormal tissue may be removed under local anaesthetic for histological examination.

The airway resistance can be measured by a technique called rhinomanometry.

Treatment of vasomotor rhinitis

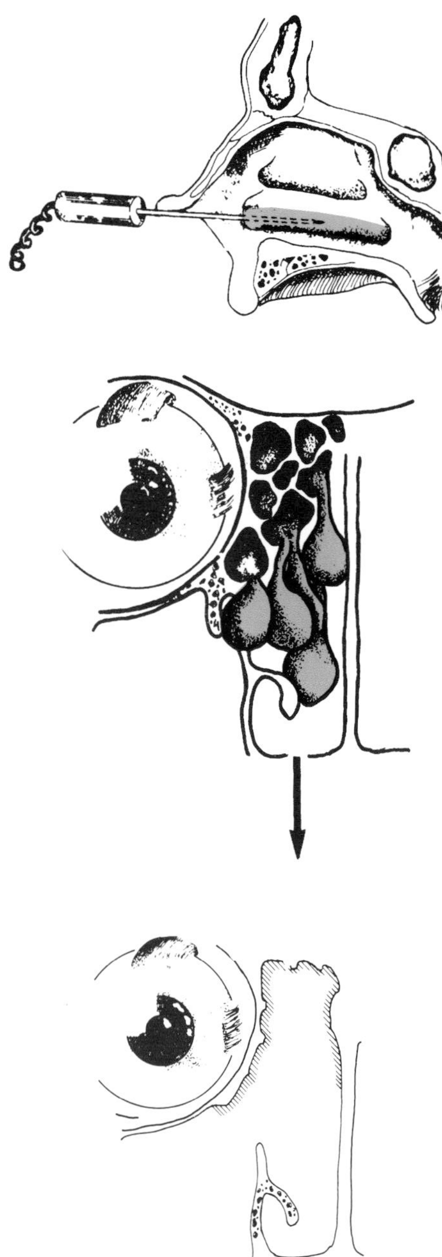

Symptomatic treatment is usually worthwhile, with antihistamines or antihistamines combined with an ephedrine-like drug in doses that do not provoke undue sleepiness. When the cause is allergic administration of a disodium cromoglycate spray may be helpful. A topical steroid spray such as beclomethasone dipropionate (Beconase) may also provide relief, again mainly for the allergic patient; it should be puffed in a dose of 50 μg to each nostril twice a day. The aqueous form is less irritating than the powder. Regular application is essential for success, and patients should be warned that the symptoms may be worse during the first few days of use. This may safely be used for long periods—certainly months—at a time. Fluticasone propionate (Flixonase) is a similar preparation for once daily use. In rare cases systemic steroids are recommended, but these should be reserved for patients with temporarily disabling symptoms, such as teenagers with hay fever faced with important examinations.

If there is no allergy, yet persistent mucosal oedema or mucosal redundancies are present one of the following operative measures may be advisable.

Submucous diathermy of the nasal mucosa is particularly helpful for children with persistently swollen inferior turbinates. Two or three strokes of the diathermy or red hot cautery needle from the back to the front of the inferior turbinates, either through or under the mucosa, will be followed by cicatricial shrinking.

Removal of nasal polyps—Single ethmoid polyps, treated for the first time, can often be removed successfully with a snare under local anaesthetic as an outpatient procedure. The aim should be to extract the polyp with the mucosa of the ethmoid cell from which it arises, rather than simply to cut it off at its neck. When polyps are numerous, sessile, or have been treated before, they should be removed under a general anaesthetic, so that the ethmoid cells from which they arise can be opened and put into continuity with each other. These "ethmoidectomies" are usually performed intranasally, but more complete clearance, with less risk of damage to the surrounding structures, such as the orbit and the anterior cranial fossa, can be achieved by an external approach through an incision around the inner canthus of the eye (external ethmoidectomy). The rare antrochoanal polyp is best treated by a Caldwell–Luc operation to expose and remove all the mucosa of the maxillary antrum from which it arises.

Moriform fringes and posterior swellings of the inferior turbinates can also be removed surgically under general anaesthetic.

A new philosophy of nasal surgery has recently emerged for the treatment of ethmoid and maxillary sinus disease. In this so called *functional endoscopic sinus surgery* the underlying principle is to restore as nearly as possible the normal functional features of the paranasal sinuses by performing very precise intranasal procedures under the magnified control of endoscopic telescopes (Hopkin's rods). The postoperative morbidity is less than with previously conventional approaches, and the techniques are being increasingly applied to allergic, vasomotor, and infective sinus disease.

Treatment of deviated nasal septum

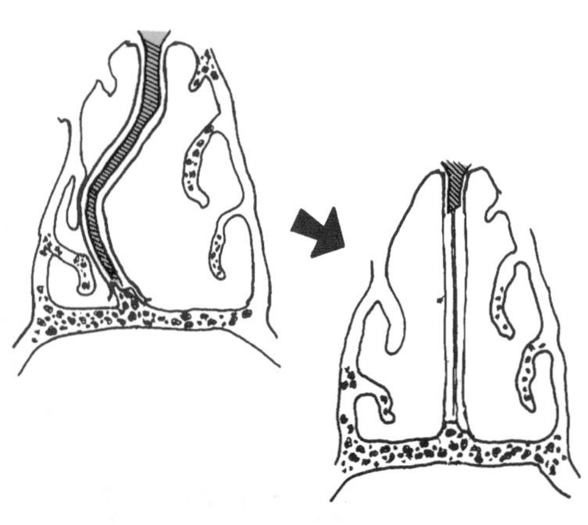

Submucous resection—A deviated nasal septum is treated by a submucous resection. This should be considered only when a deflected septum has been identified as the cause of the nasal obstruction. Submucous resection is sometimes unnecessarily performed when the main cause of obstruction is vasomotor rhinitis, and the benefits that normally follow the correct use of this operation cannot then be expected.

During the operation, which is performed under general anaesthetic, the nasal septum is "filleted" by removing the cartilage and bone that is holding the septum in the wrong position from between the layers of mucosa. The intact layers of mucosa left in contact with each other can then hang in the midline. Parts of the septal skeleton may be preserved and repositioned; the technique is called *septoplasty*. Possible complications include collapse of the nasal bridge with deformity if bridge support is lost, and perforation of the nasal septum if both layers of the mucosa are accidently transgressed.

PARANASAL SINUS DISEASES

Sinusitis

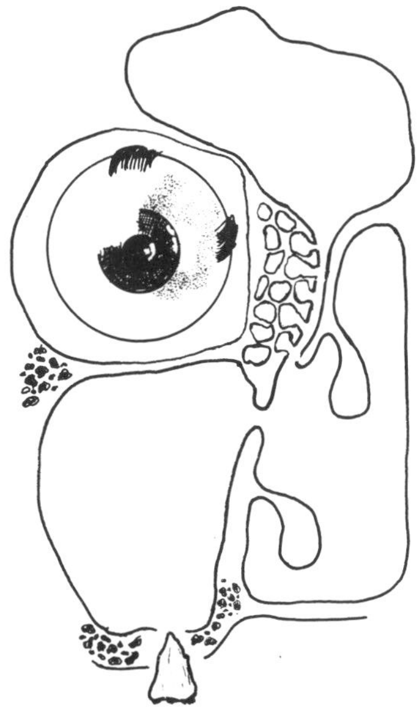

Bacterial infection of the paranasal sinuses usually occurs when the "self cleansing mechanism" becomes impaired. Mucus accumulates and stagnates within the sinus cavities and becomes infected by relatively harmless, opportunist, pyogenic bacteria normally found in the nose.

The "self cleansing mechanism" is the means whereby mucus secreted within the sinuses is swept as a continuous blanket by ciliary activity through the sinus ostia into the nose. The mucus is passed back into the nasopharynx. The process requires secretion of mucus with the correct physical characteristics; normal function of the mucosal cilia; and patency of the sinus ostia. Certain anatomical features place individual sinuses at risk: the ostium of the maxillary antrum is high on its medial wall, so mucus has to be swept upwards against gravity; the frontal sinus has a long tortuous duct, which is easily damaged and obstructed; and the ethmoid cells open into the nose in regions where they may be bathed by infected material from the maxillary sinuses.

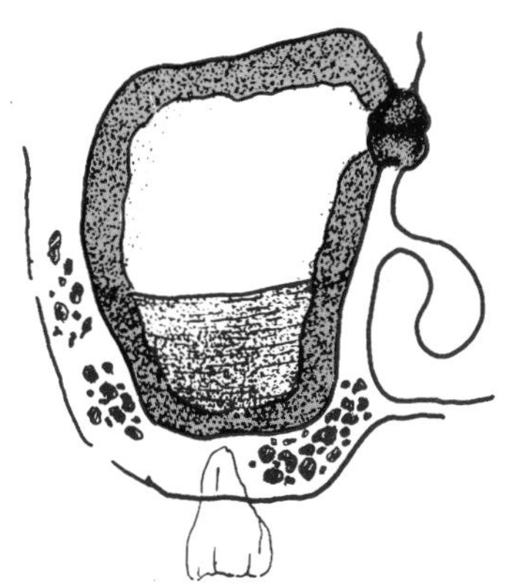

The commonest predisposing cause of derangement of self cleansing is viral infection of the nasal and sinus mucosa (viral rhinosinusitis). This depresses the activity of the cilia and provokes oedematous obstruction of the sinus ostia. Other obstructions inside the nose, including gross deflections of the nasal septum or mucosal swelling and polyps due to vasomotor rhinitis make this more likely. During a viral infection mucus accumulates in the paranasal sinuses of one or both sides. If the self cleansing mechanism does not recover the stagnating mucus becomes secondarily infected and is converted to mucopus. The mucopus impairs ciliary function, and increases the swelling around the ostia where it discharges into the nose—so creating a vicious circle.

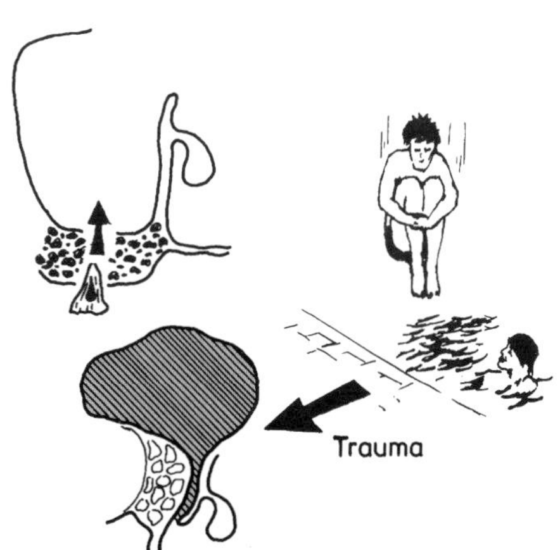

Acute sinusitis developing in this way always affects all the sinus cavities on one or both sides of the nose (pansinusitis). An individual maxillary sinus may become infected without preceding viral rhinosinusitis by direct spread of pathogenic, usually anaerobic, organisms from the tooth roots. An individual frontal sinus may become infected by traumatic inflammation of its duct caused by jumping into polluted water with the nose open.

Clinical features of sinusitis

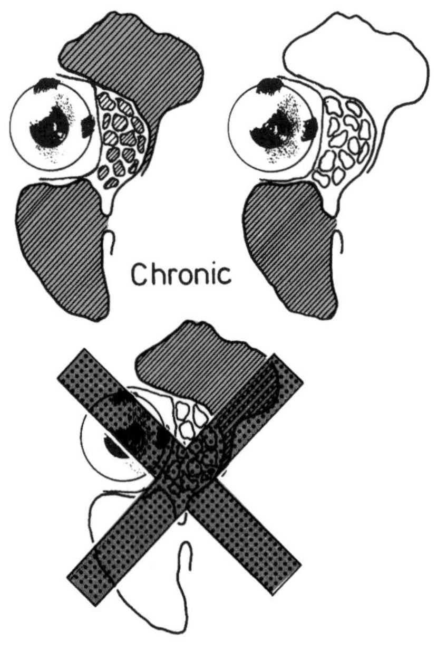

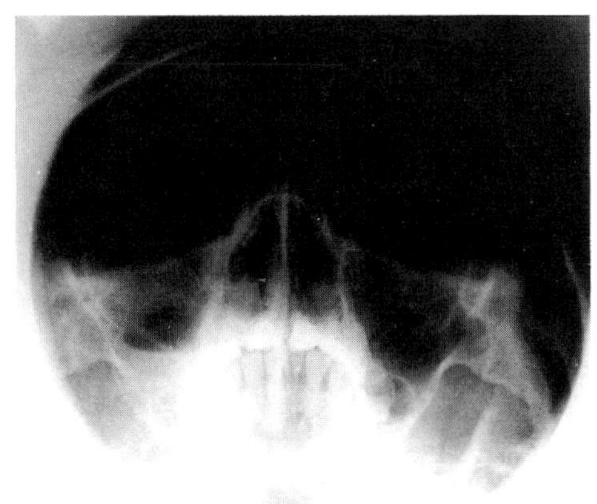

After a typical cold the symptoms do not resolve. The clear nasal discharge becomes yellow or green; fever may persist; and there is often pain in the cheek, which may be referred to the forehead. The pain becomes worse on bending or straining. If the ostium of the maxillary sinus is tightly blocked the pain may be severe and may be felt in the teeth. Tenderness is elicited by firm pressure over the maxillary antrum.

Swelling of the cheek is *never* caused by maxillary sinusitis. This symptom should suggest an infection of the root of a tooth if it is associated with an acute onset and pain, or cancer of the antrum if it is painless and develops less rapidly.

If the self cleansing mechanism fails to recover and to evacuate the mucopus after the acute illness the sinusitis enters subacute and chronic phases. Persisting chronic infection of the upper sinuses is invariably associated with infection in the lower air cells. Chronic maxillary sinusitis may exist alone, but chronic ethmoid cell infection and chronic frontal sinusitis are almost always associated with antral infection. This pattern underlies the principles of treatment.

Chronic infection is suggested by persisting nasal obstruction and purulent discharge from the nose. Pain is exceptional, but the patient may complain of dull pressure. Frontal headache is often referred from antral disease, and is caused only rarely by infection of the frontal sinus. Chronic pharyngitis and chronic laryngitis may develop.

The diagnosis is usually obvious from the history and clinical features. Examination of the interior of the nose and the nasopharynx with a mirror may show oedematous mucosa bathed in mucopus, and features such as ethmoid polyps. Radiographs are needed to confirm the diagnosis and, in chronic infection, to identify the affected sinuses.

Radiographic signs of infection are those that suggest accumulated mucopus. These are either total opacity of the affected sinus or a recognisable fluid level. The common finding of mucosal oedema within a sinus cavity must not be interpreted as evidence of infection, since this appearance, which is ephemeral, may be seen in any patient with oedema of the nasal mucosa from any cause—of which vasomotor rhinitis is the commonest. Computed tomographs, especially in the coronal plane, are more informative than conventional radiographs.

Treatment of acute sinusitis

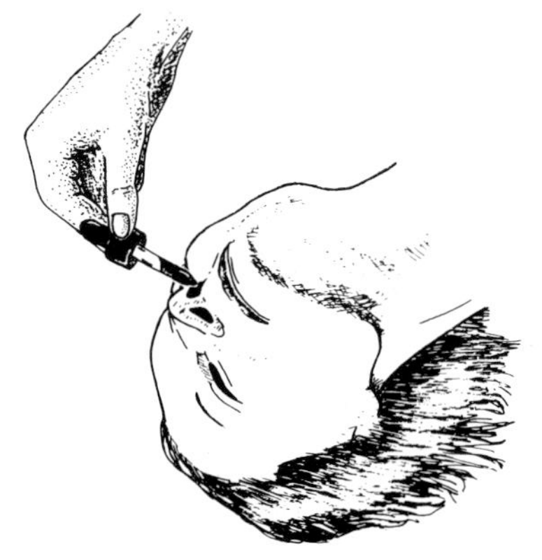

During the acute illness palliative treatment includes bedrest and analgesics. At times drugs stronger than soluble aspirin or paracetamol may be needed. Warmth from a hot water bottle may be soothing. The nasal mucosa can be decongested by using nasal drops such as ephedrine 1% in normal saline or Otrivine (xylometazoline) as drops or a spray. They should be warmed and then instilled, with the patient lying with his head over the side of the bed, breathing through his mouth. After a few drops have been instilled into each nostril, while the other is occluded, the patient should turn his head slowly from side to side for a few minutes before sitting up. Steam inhalations with benzoin tincture often help.

Bed
Analgesics
Decongestant drops
Antibiotics
Inhalations
Warmth

Systemic antibiotics are usually advisable. The choice may depend on bacteriological examination of a swab from the nasal discharge, but Vibramycin (doxycycline hydrochloride) in a daily dose of 100 mg after a loading dose of 200 mg is appropriate for adults, while penicillin or co-trimoxazole is recommended for children (though childhood sinusitis is rare).

Treatment of chronic sinusitis

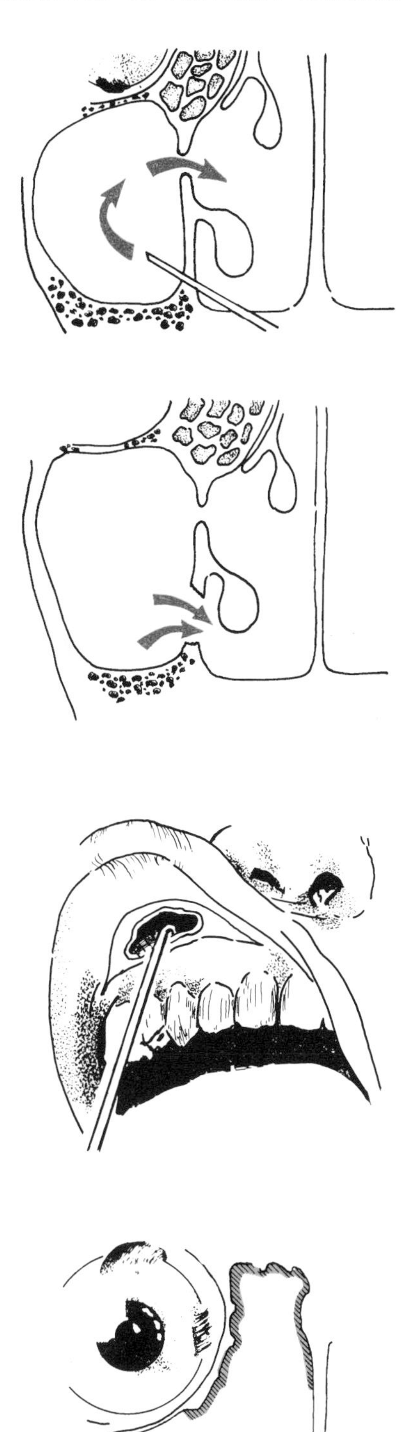

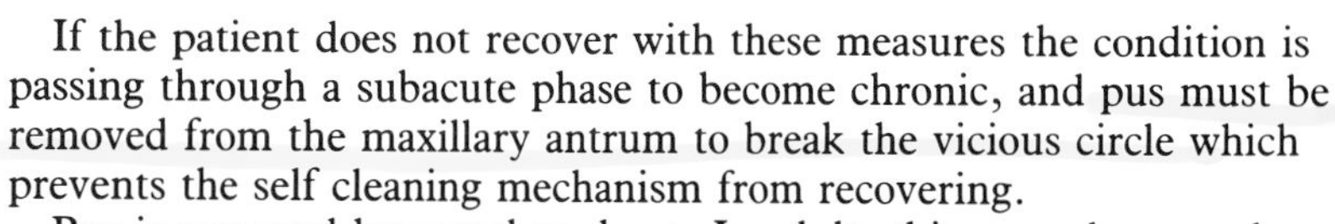

If the patient does not recover with these measures the condition is passing through a subacute phase to become chronic, and pus must be removed from the maxillary antrum to break the vicious circle which prevents the self cleaning mechanism from recovering.

Pus is removed by antral washout. In adults this procedure can be carried out under local anaesthesia by inserting a hollow cannula through the nasal wall of the maxillary antrum under the inferior turbinate. Normal saline, raised above body temperature, is instilled through the cannula by a Higginson's syringe. The contained pus and the retained fluid escape into the nose through the maxillary ostium and pour into a bowl held under the patient's chin. The patient breathes through the mouth.

Antral lavage may be needed more than once and is usually the first step in treating chronic maxillary sinusitis. Repeated antral washouts at weekly intervals are often effective in restoring normal mucosal activity (helped by the administration of a systemic antibiotic and nasal decongestants). If self cleansing recovers, the washout return will gradually change from mucopus to mucus and then to clear fluid. If the mucosa does not recover pus will be returned repeatedly, but multiple washouts are now rarely used. Very rarely, it may be necessary to drain pus from the frontal sinus during acute infection, by trephining its floor through an incision above the eye.

If maxillary sinusitis fails to respond to repeated antral lavage *intranasal antrostomy* should be considered. In this operation, performed under general anaesthetic, an additional ventilation hole is made from the maxillary sinus into the nose, as low as possible below the inferior turbinate, to allow air entry and encourage excretion of retained pus and recovery of the mucosa. *Middle meatal antrostomy*, in accordance with the principles of functional endoscopic sinus surgery (see page 42), is often now preferred to this traditional inferior meatal opening. Persisting infection after intranasal antrostomy implies that the mucosal lining is irreversibly diseased and that normal self cleansing is impossible. There may be pockets of pus inaccessible to drainage by gravity. The whole diseased lining then needs to be removed from the sinus by a *Caldwell–Luc operation* (radical antrostomy). An incision is made through the gingival mucosa within the mouth and the maxillary antrum is opened through its anterolateral wall. The antral mucosa is carefully removed and an antrostomy into the nose fashioned. This approach to the maxillary antrum may also be used to remove material for histological examination or a foreign body such as a displaced tooth root. At the end of the procedure the mucosal incision is stitched. A Caldwell–Luc operation may rarely be followed by complications such as anaesthesia or neuralgia of the infraorbital nerve.

Chronic infection in the ethmoid or frontal sinuses is treated first by eliminating infection of the maxillary antrum on that side. Treatment of persisting infection in the ethmoid labyrinth may then require an *ethmoidectomy* (as described in the chapter on nasal obstruction), particularly if polyps in the nose obstruct the ostia and prevent pus from escaping. The procedure may be carried out through the nose as an intranasal ethmoidectomy, or by external incision around the inner canthus of the eye.

Persisting frontal sinusitis can sometimes be treated by submucous resection or other minor intranasal operations to remove obstruction from the frontonasal duct. Often some form of external frontal sinus operation is needed. Many varieties are available and they rely on one of two principles. Either a new wide frontonasal duct through which infected material can escape into the nose is made, or the sinus and its duct are obliterated completely so that there is no remaining air space.

Complications of sinusitis

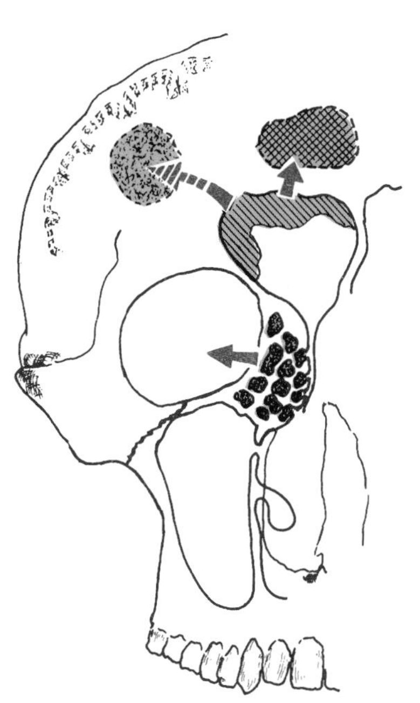

All complications of sinusitis are rare. They usually develop from infection of the ethmoid or frontal sinuses, particularly during acute exacerbations of chronic infection. Maxillary sinusitis hardly ever causes complications.

Orbital cellulitis may follow acute ethmoiditis in children or frontal sinusitis in adults. The upper eyelid becomes swollen, red, and tender, and there is associated fever. The cause can usually be recognised from the presence of pus in the nose on the affected side. If the disorder does not respond rapidly to treatment with large doses of antibiotics a subperiosteal abscess may develop within the orbit and there is a risk of damage to the eye. Computed tomography is an essential component of investigation.

Mucocoele of the frontal sinus—This complication produces swelling of the frontal sinus with erosion of the floor and displacement of the eye downwards and laterally. Swelling develops slowly and usually without pain. The patient often presents with diplopia. The condition may be identified by feeling the floor of the frontal sinus with a finger and recognising the thinning or loss of bone. The diagnosis can be confirmed by radiography. Much more rarely a mucocoele may develop in the sphenoid sinus, causing impairment of vision.

Osteomyelitis of the frontal bone is another rare but serious complication of frontal sinus disease.

Intracranial suppuration develops usually from the frontal sinus and may take the form of meningitis, extradural or subdural abscesses, or frontal lobe cerebral abscess.

Malignant tumours of the paranasal sinuses

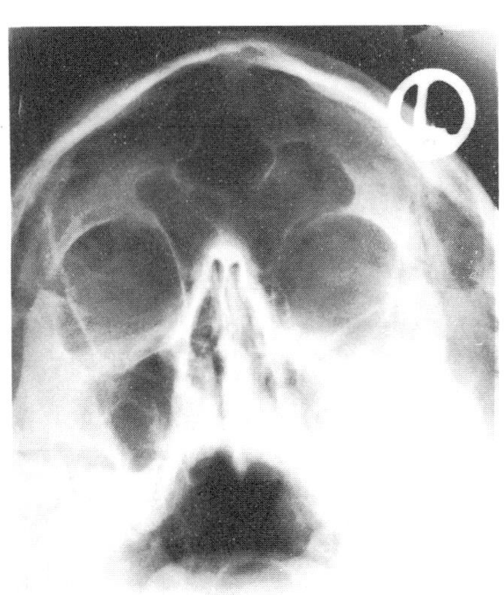

Malignant tumours of the paranasal sinuses are almost always squamous cell carcinomas and usually develop in middle aged or elderly men. Neoplasia should be suspected in any patient who develops chronic sinusitis for the first time in later life without an obvious cause. Extension beyond the bony walls of the ethmoid or maxillary sinuses causes swelling of the face; displacement of the eye with proptosis and diplopia; nasal obstruction and blood stained discharge; and swelling of the palate or loosening of teeth. Any of these symptoms is highly suggestive. Apart from the swelling, there may be friable vascular material in the nasal cavity, from which a biopsy specimen must be taken. Radiography with tomography will almost always show erosion of bone. A Caldwell–Luc operation may be needed to provide material for histological examination. These tumours hardly ever spread to regional lymph nodes. Treatment includes radiotherapy, radical surgical removal, and cytotoxic chemotherapy.

NOSE BLEEDS

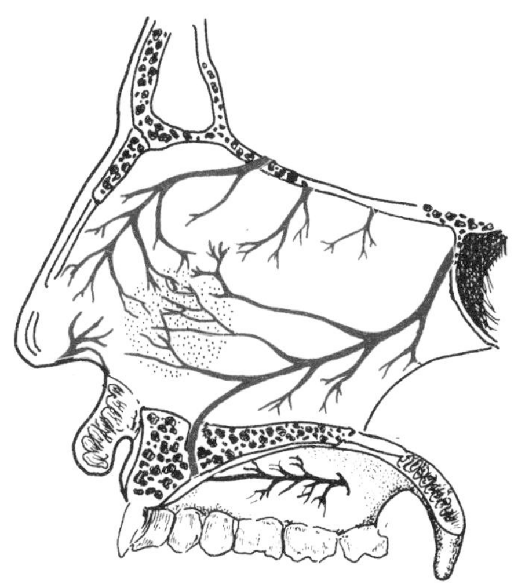

Most nose bleeds come from ruptured blood vessels on the nasal septum. In young people the bleeding is usually from a vein just behind the columella. In older patients the bleeding is arterial, from the caudal part of the nasal septum, where there is a region of multiple arterial anastomosis—Little's area. In both groups the cause may be unrecognised, or the bleeding may be due to minimal trauma from sneezing or nose blowing. In elderly patients arterial bleeding is often associated with degenerative arterial disease and hypertension. Rarer causes include clotting defects in blood dyscrasias; local vascular malformations in hereditary telangiectasia; raised venous blood pressure (either generalised in congestive heart failure or localised in superior mediastinal obstruction).

Management

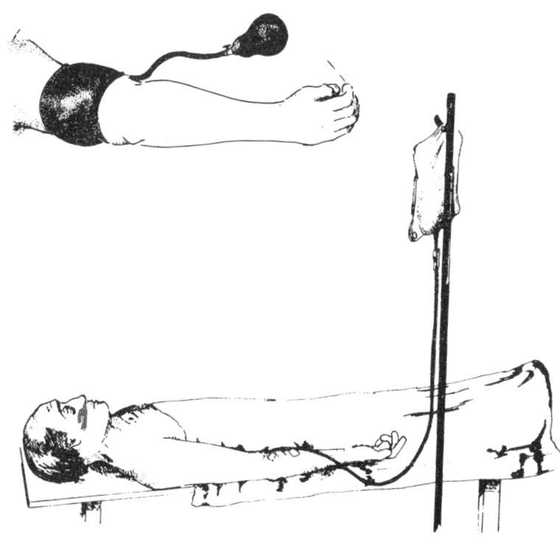

The doctor must (*a*) assess the effects of blood loss and, if necessary, replace blood by transfusion; (*b*) identify the source of bleeding within the nose and try to find the cause; and (*c*) stop the bleeding.

The effects of blood loss must be assessed before any effort is made to find the source of bleeding and to stop it. An elderly patient who has lost a lot of blood is more likely to die during the next few hours from the effects of the blood loss already sustained than from the results of continuing bleeding. Clinical assessment, including pulse and blood pressure measurements, will indicate whether the patient is shocked. If so a blood sample should immediately be taken for grouping and cross matching and intravenous infusion with a plasma expander started.

The position of the patient is important. It is often suggested that a patient with a bleeding nose should be nursed upright to lower the venous blood pressure. That may be useful advice for a young, fit patient who has lost a little blood from the nose; but any patient who has suffered extensive blood loss must be kept with the head low to maintain an adequate circulation to the brain.

When the doctor is happy about the patient's general condition, as is usually so on first acquaintance with a young patient, attention can turn to the source of trouble—the bleeding nose.

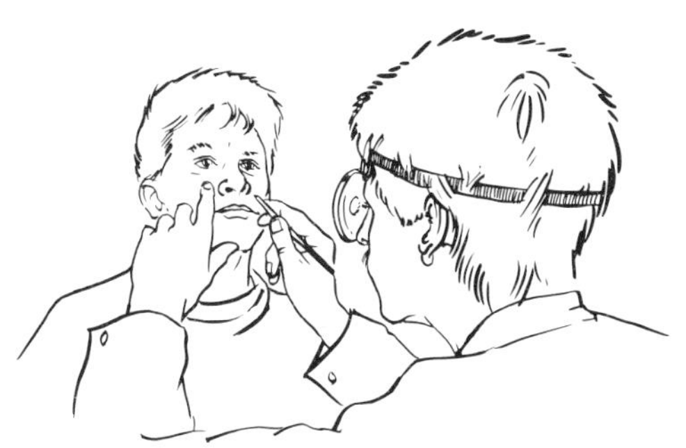

First aid measures

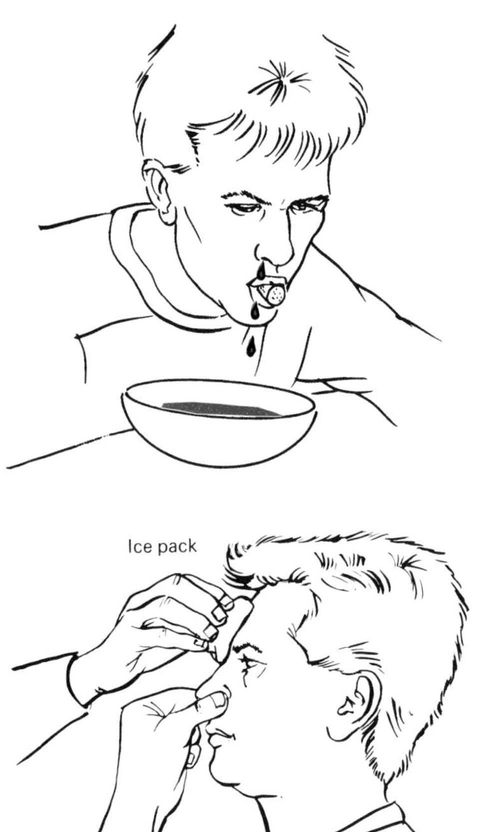

The patient himself may be able to stop bleeding from the anterior part of the nose by pinching the nostril between a finger and thumb and applying ice packs to the bridge of the nose. If this is not effective then he should sit down and hold a bowl into which the blood can drip. Swallowing, which would displace the accumulating clot, must be discouraged. It can be prevented most easily by placing a cork between the teeth (Trotter's method).

The doctor should sit the patient, if fit enough, opposite. Ideally illumination should be with a headlight so that both hands can be free. Clotted blood should be removed from the nose with either Luc's forceps or a sucker. As each part of the nasal mucosa comes into view it may be sprayed with cocaine solution (2·5–10%). This helps to stop the bleeding by constricting the blood vessels and it anaesthetises the mucosa so that any later manoeuvre can be performed without discomfort. As clot removal and spraying proceed alternately the nasal interior becomes visible. If no headlight is available the doctor may have to pack the nose "blindly" with ribbon gauze (see below).

The next measures depend on whether the bleeding has stopped and what has been found in the nose.

If the nose is clear and the bleeding stops no local treatment is needed. The patient should be watched for a while to make sure there is no further bleeding, and bed rest with sedation may be recommended.

If the bleeding continues and the bleeding point is visible the vessels can be cauterised. This is done, after anaesthetising the mucosa with cocaine, by touching the site with a bead of silver nitrate on a stick, a cotton wool probe moistened in trichloracetic acid, or the point of a red hot electrocautery point.

If the bleeding continues and no source can be found it must be controlled by the pressure of a pack in the nose.

Packing the nose

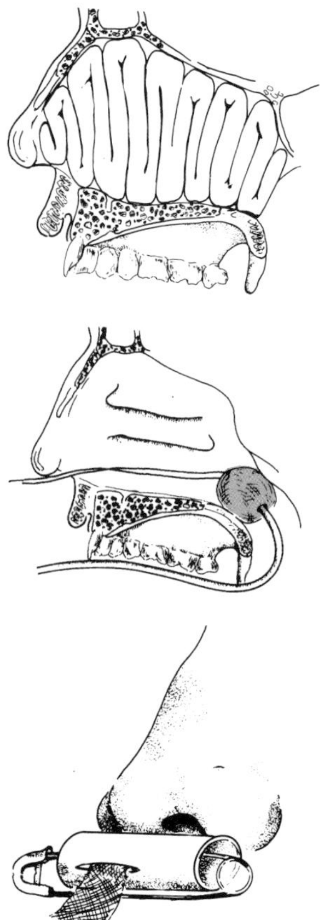

An anterior nasal pack of ribbon gauze fills the nose from the front. The gauze ($\frac{1}{2}$ in or 1 in) is moistened with paraffin or bismuth subnitrate and iodoform paste (BIPP) and inserted with Tilley's nasal dressing forceps. The patient may safely be allowed to return home, and the pack may be left undisturbed for two or three days.

Posterior nasal pack—If bleeding continues despite the presence of an effective anterior nasal pack, pressure on the walls of the postnasal space is needed. A posterior pack is made from a wadge of gauze as large as the end of the patient's thumb, which is rammed tightly into the posterior choana. The gauze has two firmly attached tapes and is moistened with paraffin or BIPP to hinder infection and to lubricate. This pack has to be inserted with local anaesthesia of the nose and throat or, in some cases, under a general anaesthetic. A thin rubber catheter is passed into the nose from the front until its tip reaches the throat. The end is found at the back of the throat by inspection and is drawn out of the mouth with a pair of forceps. One of the tapes attached to the pack is tied to the end of the catheter. The catheter is then withdrawn from the nose so that it pulls first the tape and then the pack into the postnasal space. A finger must guide the tape around the soft palate to prevent abrasion. The nasal tape is then fastened (as shown) so that it pulls the pack firmly into the back of the nose and its loose end is strapped to the cheek. The mouth tape, which will be used to withdraw the pack, is loosely strapped to the cheek, taking care that it does not cut the corner of the mouth. A patient with a postnasal pack in place must stay in hospital. The postnasal pack should be removed after 24 hours because of the risks of infection and damage to the orifice of the Eustachian tube.

Continued bleeding after packing

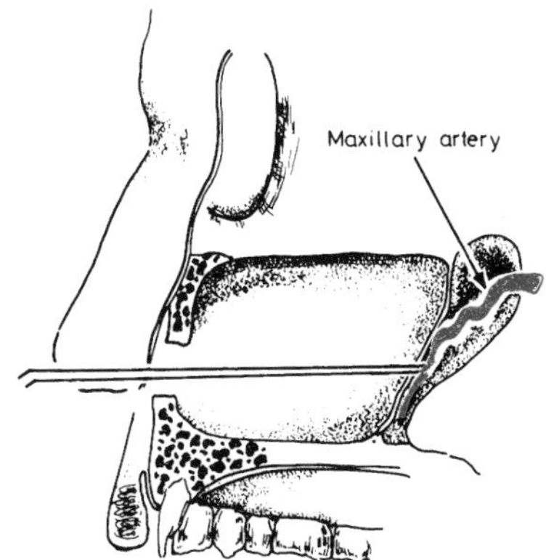

After removing nasal packs there may be no further bleeding, but bleeding often starts again, either at once or a few hours later. For this reason a patient should not be discharged from care immediately. Repeated bleeding may be controlled by repeated packing. Unfortunately, nasal packing, particularly of the postnasal space, is extremely uncomfortable and if prolonged and repeated the patient becomes miserable and the surgeon dispirited. Continued bleeding after removal of a second or third set of packs is best managed by ligating the arterial supply to the nose. The main source of this supply is from the maxillary artery—a branch of the external carotid artery. A minor contribution is from the anterior ethmoidal artery—a source ultimately derived from the internal carotid.

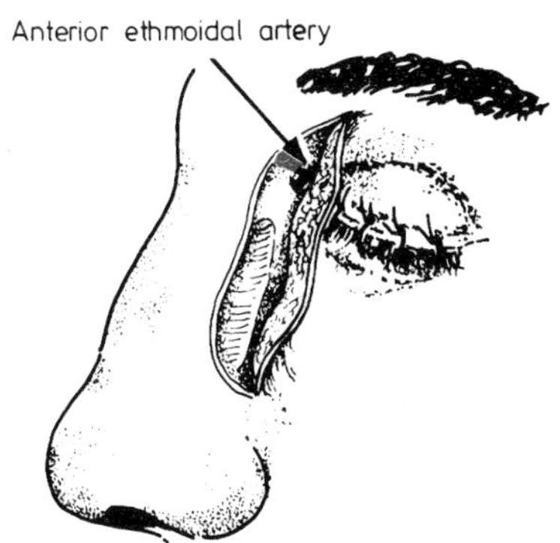

The anterior ethmoidal artery is accessible through an incision around the inner canthus of the eye on the medial wall of the orbit, but since it provides only a small contribution to the blood supply of the nose, it is usually better to ligate one of the other vessels, regardless of the site of the bleeding. For the general surgeon the external carotid artery, approached in the neck, is the obvious choice. For the otolaryngologist ligation or clipping of the maxillary artery in the pterygopalatine fossa is easily achieved, by a Caldwell–Luc approach to and through the posterior wall of the antrum.

Very rarely bleeding may continue despite these measures. Ligation of the other vessel is then usually recommended. As a last resort low doses of radiotherapy to the nasal mucosa may be effective.

INJURIES AND FOREIGN BODIES

Injuries to the nose

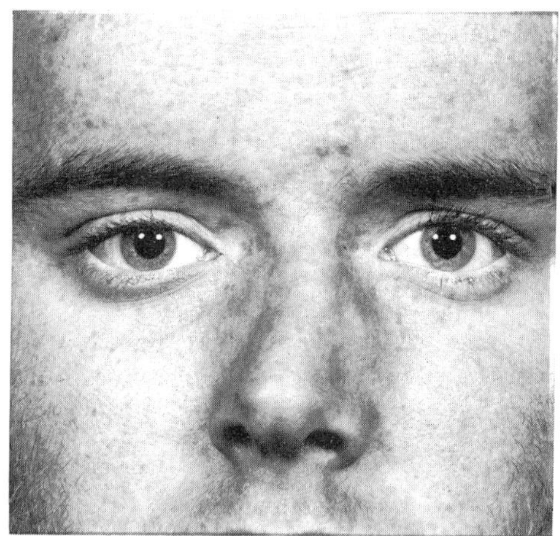

Fractured nasal bones—Direct violence to the nose often fractures the bones of the nasal vault. The injury can usually be recognised clinically immediately afterwards by the distortion from normal shape, though this soon becomes obscured by soft tissue swelling.

Injuries to other parts of the facial skeleton must be excluded: associated fractures of the zygomaticomaxillary complex may impair normal opening of the jaw and cause faulty dental occlusion, diplopia, and anaesthesia of the skin supplied by the infraorbital nerve. These injuries are always associated with rapid swelling of the soft tissues of the cheek, and a subconjunctival haemorrhage is usually apparent. Careful palpation of the bony skeleton around the edge of the orbit may disclose a typical "step" deformity.

Management of nasal injuries

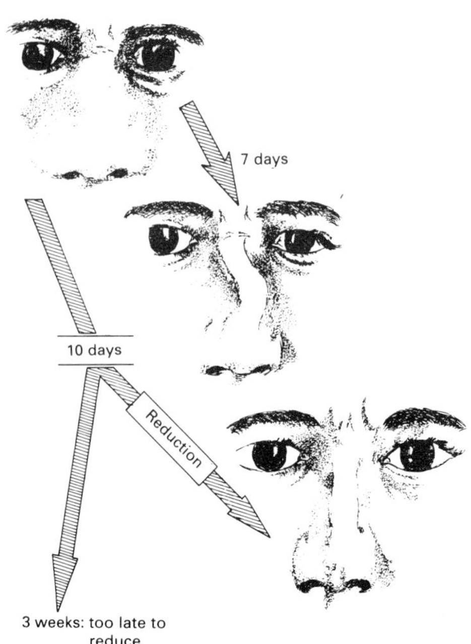

Radiographs of the nose are not usually needed to establish the diagnosis of a fracture or the need for treatment, but are often performed for medicolegal reasons. Fractures of the nasal vault require surgical reduction only when there is deformity. It is often difficult to assess the deviation from normal shape until the soft tissue swelling has subsided, which may take five to seven days. Since the nasal bones will become firmly set within three weeks of the injury, the need for treatment should be assessed after a week, and, if necessary, reduction under general anaesthetic should be planned for the following week. Fractures of the zygoma and maxilla set firmly very much more quickly—within a few days. If a zygomaticomaxillary fracture is suspected the patient should therefore be referred to a faciomaxillary surgeon immediately.

Nasal injuries often cause deflection of the nasal septum with obstruction of the nose. This can rarely be corrected satisfactorily at the time of reducing a nasal fracture, and the deflection is best treated by submucous resection several months later.

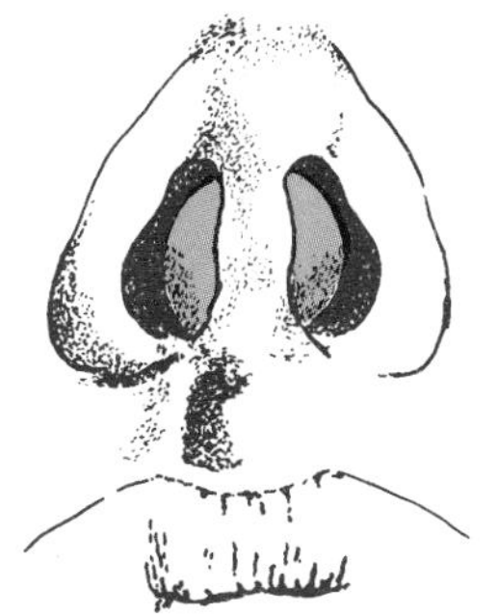

Septal haematoma may occur after injury to the nose. This causes total nasal obstruction and is easily recognised as gross swelling of both sides of the nasal septum visible from the front of the nose. Urgent treatment is needed to prevent the development of a septal abscess, which may lead to necrosis of the cartilaginous structure of the nose followed by collapse and unsightly deformity. The blood clot should be removed through an incision, under local anaesthetic, and the patient given systemic antibiotics.

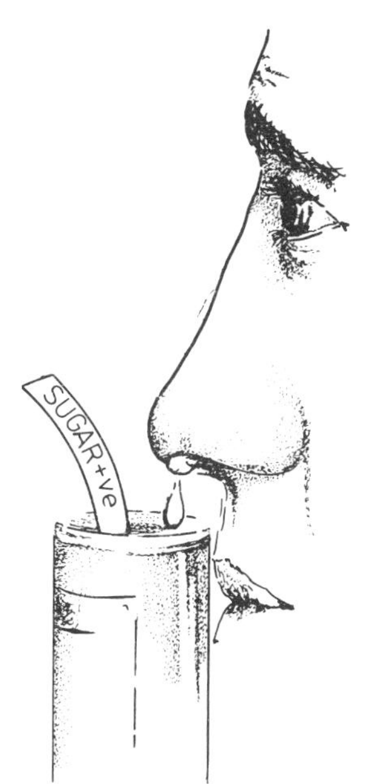

CSF rhinorrhoea—Nasal injuries may be associated with cerebrospinal fluid rhinorrhoea from a fracture of the roof of the ethmoid labyrinth into the anterior cranial fossa. If this is suspected the patient should be warned not to blow his nose and to remain in a sitting position. A collection of fluid dripping from the nose should be tested biochemically—first for the presence of reducing sugars, which would suggest that the fluid is CSF. Although CSF rhinorrhoea may cease spontaneously, it is common practice to recommend neurosurgical closure of a possible defect in the dura to prevent subsequent attacks of meningitis. Loss of the sense of smell is another sequel to nasal injuries and also to head injuries in which swivelling of the brain within the skull tears the roots of the olfactory nerve. There is no treatment. Rarely, fractures of the ethmoid are followed by surgical emphysema at the side of the nose. This develops when the nose is blown and the characteristic crepitus is always obvious on palpating the swelling. Although alarming the condition needs no special treatment.

Chronic damage to the nasal septum by picking the nose or by inhaling irritants such as cocaine may eventually cause perforation of the septum. Septal perforations create a feeling of discomfort and of nasal obstruction. Crusts that develop around the edges of the perforation separate from time to time, damage the septal mucosa, and so enlarge the perforation.

Injuries to the ear

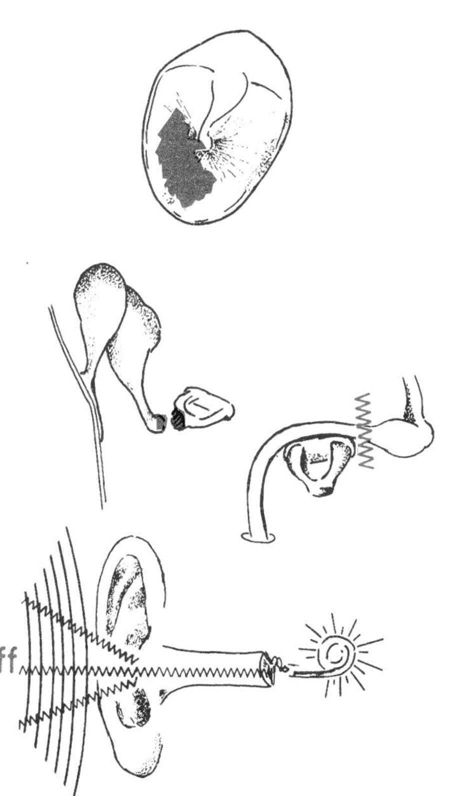

Blows to the pinna may cause haematomas, which, if untreated, may result in cauliflower ears. The accumulated blood should either be aspirated through a wide bore needle or evacuated through an incision. Injuries of the tympanic membrane and middle ear have been discussed in the chapter on pain in the ear. There is rarely any urgent need to assess either the state of the drum or hearing. Blood clot obscuring the meatus may safely be left to separate itself; then the ear may be examined fully. The patient should be warned to keep water out of the ear in case the tympanic membrane is perforated. Damage to the drum or the ossicular chain found later can often be corrected surgically. Facial palsy developing from an injury to the ear is usually a sequal to a fracture of the petrous temporal bone. If there is any doubt about the continuity of the nerve surgical exploration may be needed. Cerebrospinal fluid otorrhoea sometimes follows fractures to the base of the skull. Leaks usually cease spontaneously after two to three weeks, in which case no further attention is necessary.

Injuries to the ear by barotrauma have been discussed in the chapter on pain in the ear and those caused by noise to the cochlea in the chapter on deafness in adults.

Foreign bodies in the nose

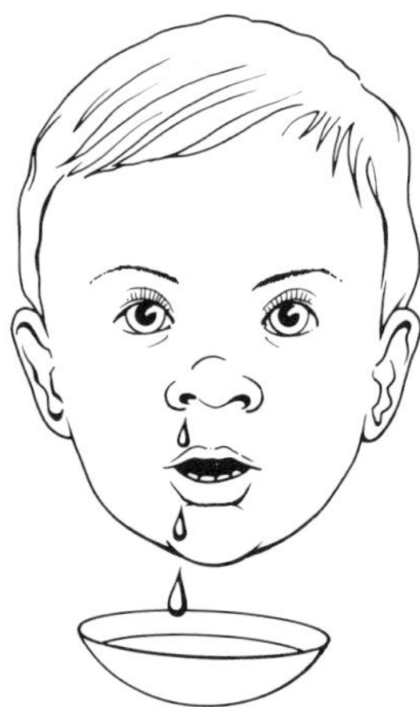

Most foreign bodies in the nose are inserted intentionally by children. Inert mineral foreign bodies may remain in place causing no symptoms for long periods, and their insertion may not be suspected unless a careful inventory is made of each component of every toy before tidying up at night. Organic foreign bodies such as pieces of apple, fragments of toilet paper, or bits of sponge produce an inflammatory reaction with purulent discharge. Unilateral purulent nasal discharge always indicates a foreign body in the nose. Armed with this suspicion and a pair of Tilley's forceps, the doctor should inspect the nose with a headlight. The foreign body may often be seized and removed with the forceps before the child is aware of the assault. If this is not possible it is useful to spray the nasal mucosa with 2.5% cocaine. The ensuing mucosal shrinkage may allow expulsion of the foreign body by blowing the nose or ease its extraction with a sucker. Some hard objects such as beads may be rolled along the floor of the nose with a blunt hook. If any difficulty is encountered with an uncooperative child general anaesthesia will be necessary and care must be taken to protect the airway from displacement of the foreign body into the nasopharynx.

Foreign bodies in the ear

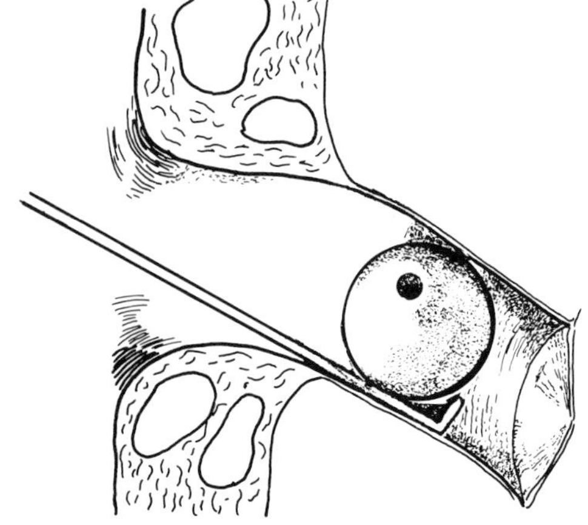

Foreign bodies in the ear are also usually inserted intentionally by children or mentally disturbed adults. Unless removal is likely to be successful at the first attempt the child should be referred for expert specialist attention, since unsuccessful attempts at removal may push the object further into the meatus and damage the drum and middle ear. General anaesthesia is often needed and even then extraction of hard slippery items can be difficult.

Inhaled foreign bodies

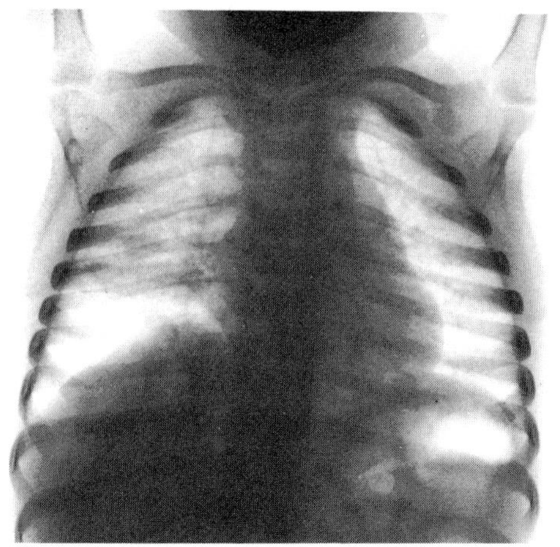

The reactions produced by foreign bodies in the tracheobronchial tree depend on their nature. Vegetable foreign bodies excite a vigorous inflammatory reaction, with purulent bronchitis and sometimes collapse of a lobe of the lung. There may also be obstructive emphysema. Mineral foreign bodies produce much less reaction and are easily overlooked. The sudden onset of stridor, cough, or dyspnoea in a previously healthy patient should suggest the possibility of a foreign body. Unilateral wheezing is particularly suspicious. Removal requires the skilled attention of a bronchoscopist, and many foreign bodies are now extracted with a fibreoptic bronchoscope under local anaesthetic.

Swallowed foreign bodies

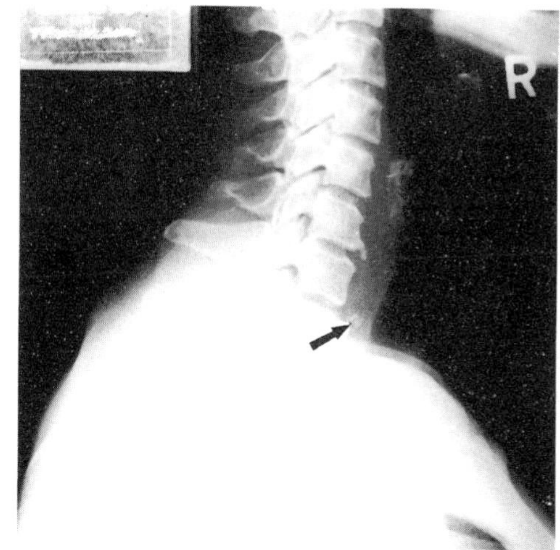

Small, sharp foreign bodies such as fish bones often stick in the lower pole of the tonsils. They may be found by careful examination with a headlight and may often be removed using a tongue depressor in one hand and a pair of Luc's forceps in the other. A suspicion that fish bones are impacted below that level may be confirmed by the laryngologist using a laryngeal mirror for indirect laryngoscopy. It may sometimes be possible to remove a bone from there under inspection with a laryngeal mirror, without general anaesthesia. Foreign bodies in the oesophagus usually impact at the upper end, just below the cricopharyngeus. Occasionally they may be obstructed by a stricture. Most common are coins, bones, and lumps of meat. These are more likely to be ingested by patients with dentures and those who gulp their food.

Pain on swallowing
Pain in ear
Tenderness in neck
Fever

It is not always easy to confirm or refute a patient's belief that he has a foreign body stuck in the gullet. A sensation of sharp pain on swallowing is very suspicious, especially if it radiates to the ear. Difficulty in swallowing saliva and tenderness in the neck or tenderness on pressure over the trachea are suspicious physical signs. Fever, developing some hours after the incident, suggests the possibility of perforation of the oesophageal wall. After the first day increasing pain is a worrying feature.

Radiographs of the neck and chest often show nothing abnormal. Many foreign bodies, particularly fish bones and some dental plates, are radiolucent. Occasionally surgical emphysema is seen as an air shadow in the prevertebral tissues, indicating rupture of the oesophagus. If a sharp foreign body might be impacted the patient should be admitted to hospital. Slender evidence may justify observation for 12 hours or so to see whether the symptoms abate.

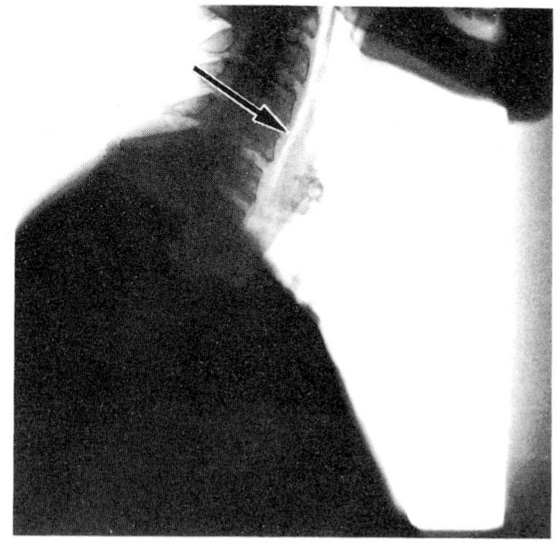

Under all other circumstances oesophagoscopy to find and remove the foreign body is necessary. Barium swallow beforehand is usually undesirable since the barium in the oesophagus will make examination more difficult and may provoke problems with the anaesthetic. Some foreign bodies, particularly open safety pins and dentures with metal hooks, present difficult, dangerous problems and there is a risk of rupturing the oesophagus during extraction. After any oesophagoscopy the patient must be watched carefully for signs that might suggest a breach of the oesophageal wall—increasing pain or tenderness in the neck, fever, or radiological evidence of surgical emphysema.

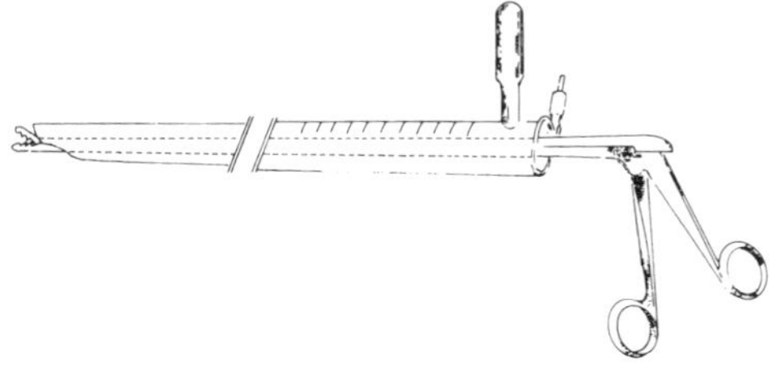

INDEX

Index